John Henry Steel

A treatise on the diseases of the dog;

Being a manual of canine pathology. Especially adapted for the use of veterinary practitioners and students

John Henry Steel

A treatise on the diseases of the dog;
Being a manual of canine pathology. Especially adapted for the use of veterinary practitioners and students

ISBN/EAN: 9783337814960

Printed in Europe, USA, Canada, Australia, Japan

Cover: Foto ©ninafisch / pixelio.de

More available books at **www.hansebooks.com**

A TREATISE

ON THE

DISEASES OF THE DOG;

BEING A

MANUAL OF CANINE PATHOLOGY.

ESPECIALLY ADAPTED FOR THE USE OF VETERINARY
PRACTITIONERS AND STUDENTS.

BY

JOHN HENRY STEEL, M.R.C.V.S., A.V.D.,

PROFESSOR OF VETERINARY SCIENCE AND SUPERINTENDENT, BOMBAY
VETERINARY COLLEGE;
LATE DEMONSTRATOR OF AND LECTURER ON ANATOMY AT THE
ROYAL VETERINARY COLLEGE OF LONDON;
CORRESPONDING MEMBER OF THE ITALIAN VETERINARY ACADEMY;
AUTHOR OF 'OUTLINES OF EQUINE ANATOMY,' 'DISEASES
OF THE ELEPHANT,' 'BOVINE PATHOLOGY;' AND
CO-EDITOR OF THE 'QUARTERLY JOURNAL OF VETERINARY SCIENCE IN
INDIA.'

NEW YORK:
JOHN WILEY & SONS, 15, ASTOR PLACE.
1888.

To

SIR DINSHAW MANOCKJEE PETIT, Kt.,

SHERIFF OF THE CITY OF BOMBAY;

WHOSE

LARGE-HEARTED LIBERALITY HAS, AMONG NUMEROUS FORMS

OF BENEFACTION, FOUND EXPRESSION IN THE

ESTABLISHMENT OF THE

BAI SAKARBAI DINSHAW PETIT HOSPITAL FOR ANIMALS,

THIS WORK,

WHICH ALSO AIMS AT ALLEVIATION OF THE ILLS THE FLESH

OF LOWER ANIMALS IS HEIR TO, IS DEDICATED

BY THE FIRST SUPERINTENDENT OF

THAT HOSPITAL,

THE AUTHOR.

PREFACE.

This book has its origin in the feeling that though since the days of Blaine and Youatt there have been many writers on canine pathology, the true bearings and progress of that science have not been dealt with so systematically and thoroughly as is needed to meet the requirements of the present day. As canine practice is more and more coming into the hands of veterinary surgeons, the want of a modern systematic text-book has become more felt, and it is to meet this want the author has prepared the following chapters. The enormous amount of valuable material contained in English periodical literature has been carefully studied, the work of leading veterinarians on the Continent has been laid under contribution, and the author has not failed to consult all available British authorities in the interests of his readers; thus it is hoped that the combined experience of the British and foreign canine pathologists will be found condensed in this work, digested, arranged, and "steadied" by the author's not inconsiderable experience of diseases of the dog and of the specialties of canine practice.

It is for the profession to determine whether the aims of this work have been carried out; it has been hoped to continue the systematic arrangement, careful record of personal observations, and constant eye to comparative study of BLAINE, with the thorough collection and digest of

PAGE

croton oil, Epsom salts, castor-oil, cathartic mixture. Preparation for physic. *Emetics:* salt with mustard is a common emetic, tartar emetic, calomel. *Vermifuges:* areca nut, oil of turpentine, santonin, calomel, kousso, hellebore, filix mas. *Stimulants, Sedatives, and Narcotics:* opium; differences between the action of certain agents on the dog and on man; chloroform. *Anæsthetics:* administration; Gruby on the effects of ether on dogs. Relation of doses for dogs to those for horses. Subcutaneous injection of medicines. *External Applications and Minor Surgery:* blisters, firing, setons, fomentations; baths, warm, cold; washing, bleeding, rough means for local bleeding; bandaging, muzzling. Leading differences between canine and veterinary surgery . 14—25

CHAPTER III.—DISEASES OF THE BLOOD.

General remarks. SPECIFIC DISORDERS: RABIES. Its importance in relation to public health. Symptoms to be studied only in relation to diagnosis. Liability of owners for acts of dogs known to be mad. Diagnosis. Varieties of the disorder. Bouley's rule. Excessive affection suspicious. Fury. Escape and journeying. Attack. The water fallacy. Peculiar expression, especially in the dumb form. Bone-in-the-throat fallacy. State of appetite. Influence of sex. The eye of a mad dog. Digestive and sexual derangements. Alteration in voice. Local irritation. Blaine's views on temporary localisation of the virus. Post-mortem diagnosis. Mistake in prompt slaughter of a dog which has bitten a man. Incubation. Lesions of alimentary and respiratory organs. Of nervous centra. Accessory observations. The eye changes in rabies by Siedamgrotzsky. On the minute changes of the nerve-centres, by Coats, Gowers, and Kolessnikow. Pasteur's researches on the virulence of the substance of nerve-centra. Diagnostic inoculation of rabies to rabbits and birds. The differential diagnosis of rabies; popular errors; distemper, fits, canker of the ear, tetanus, &c. Appliances for seizure of mad dog. Prophylaxis. Means of conveyance of the disease. Post-mortem examinations, precautions in. Destruction of carcass. Curative treatment unsuccessful. Possibility of fortifying the constitution against it not unlikely. Pasteurean system of rabies' inoculation. Extermination of dogs (note on skunk bite), dogs' homes, quarantine, and other measures of repression, valuable but limited in efficacy. Breed most liable to convey the disease. Muzzling. Bourrel's operation of blunting the teeth. Measures in case of actual infliction of a bite by a mad dog. If the patient be a dog and has not since bitten a man. Chances of the animal not developing the disease after a bite. Measures to be taken when a human being has been bitten. Difficult double duty of the canine pathologist in dealing with rabies. DISTEMPER: its fatality, specificity, prevalence, and invasion. Its relations to similar disorders of other species. Semmer's bacterium. Effects of the poison on the blood. Types. Predisposing causes. Supposed spontaneous origin. Differential diagnosis. Symptoms: General; eye ulceration. Prognosis. Nervous sequelæ. Intestinal form. Respiratory and hepatic forms. Skin eruption. Post-mortem appearances by Semmer. Treatment. Disinfection and measures against contagion not sufficiently enforced. Blaine's "virulent or putrid type." Medicinal treatment. Debilitating measures to be specially avoided. Nursing tonics. Persistency apt to be rewarded. DIPHTHERIA: Robertson's outbreak. Structural alterations. Three types: first, second, third or nasal. Sequelæ. Opinions of Law and Bossi on this subject; the latter records a case of conveyance from a child to a dog. Letzerich on vaccination of a dog with lymph containing diphtheritic material. ECZEMA EPIZOOTICA: occurs in dog. Pallin's case in a cat. RELAPSING FEVER, "SURRA." ANTHRAX: not frequent in carnivora. Intestinal form most frequent, its causes and symptoms. Post-mortem appearances. Rougieux' account of an outbreak in fox-hounds. Toussaint's conclusions concerning anthrax vaccination of dogs. The liability of dogs to anthrax in the form of blebs or pustules in the mouth. Conveyance of the disease *by the bite*. VARIOLA CANINA rare. Its relations to smallpox and Var. ovina. *Malignant* or *Benign*. Symptoms. Treatment. "Unicity" of this disease. Influence of heat and cold on its development. GLANDERS: Lafosse, Polli, Renault, Hertwig, St. Cyr, and Nordström on its conveyance to dogs. MEASLES: a case of fatal communication from a child. CHOLERA: Surgeon-Major Fairweather's Report on the cat epizooty at Delhi. TUBERCULOSIS. Does true "consumption" occur in the dog? Colin and Laulanié on false pulmonary tubercle due to parasites. Nodular disease apparently tubercular. Causes. Heredity. Breeding errors. Tabes. Symptoms. Bowel and lung cases. Treatment. Gowing on scrofulous change of the liver. SEPTICÆMIA: especially frequent in parturient bitches. Symptoms and post-mortem appearances. NON-SPECIFIC DISORDERS: RHEUMATISM. Frequent in sporting dogs. Causes. Acute or chronic. Richardson's experiment on the artificial production of rheumatism. Special features of this disease in the dog. *Lumbago*. *Chest founder* and *Kennel lameness*. Youatt's views. Treatment of the chronic and acute forms. Prevention. RICKETS: M. Voit's experimental study of the disease. Hill's remarks. Symptoms and differential diagnosis. Treatment. LEUKÆMIA: its study by Siedamgrotzsky. Three forms. Autopsy. Diagnosis. Innorenza's views. JAUNDICE or ICTERUS: Causes. "*The Yellows.*" Symptoms. Treatment. Special liability of the dog to nutritive defects. ANÆMIA. PLETHORA: "*Foul*" (Mayhew). FEVER: Simple, Malarious. Obscurity of such cases . . 26—72

CHAPTER IV.—DISEASES OF THE CIRCULATORY SYSTEM.

INTRODUCTION. Simplicity of the organs. Deficiency in records of disease of them. Heart. FIBROUS DEPOSITS ON THE VALVES. FATTY DEGENERATION OF THE HEART. RUPTURE OF THE HEART WALLS. DISEASES OF THE PERICARDIUM. Punctured wound of the pericardium and walls of the chest. CANINE HÆMATOZOA: *Filaria immitis*. WORM IN THE HEART. Manson's researches. Diagnosis. Tuberculoid disease of the lungs as a sequela. Symptoms. Hollingham's case. *Filaria sanguinolenta*. Observations by Dr. Lewis of Calcutta. Dr. Manson's views. Autopsy. Manson on the effects of these worms as causing stricture of œsophagus, pleurisy, and paraplegia. Relations of these worms to hæmatozoa of man. Supposed source of the parasites. *Congenital malformation* of pre-caval veins in the dog . . . . . 73—81

CHAPTER V.—DISEASES OF THE RESPIRATORY SYSTEM.

INTRODUCTION. Variation according to breed—the acute, degenerative, and parasitic. *Nasal chambers and their accessories;* their anatomy and physiology. CATARRH or CORYZA. SORE-THROAT. OZŒNA. PARASITIC OZŒNA due to pentastomes. POLYPUS IN THE NOSTRILS: *Snorting, Epistaxis*. DISEASES OF THE AIR PASSAGES: Preliminary remarks on anatomy and physiology. COUGH (*Acute and Chronic*), *Loss of voice, Snoring,* ACUTE LARYNGITIS, *Laryngismus stridulus, Chronic laryngitis*. Mayhew's caution as to insertion of seton in the throat. *Of the essential organs of Respiration :* anatomy, auscultation, percussion, succussion, measurement. INFLAMMATION OF THE ORGANS IN THE CHEST, *i.e.* BRONCHITIS, PNEUMONIA, AND PLEURISY, and their complications. Causes. Symptoms. HYDROTHORAX: Blaine on diagnosis of this affection. Treatment. Paracentesis thoracis. VERMINOUS BRONCHITIS: Osler's researches. ASTHMA or CHRONIC BRONCHITIS: Congestive and spasmodic . . 82—97

CHAPTER VI.—DISORDERS OF THE DIGESTIVE APPARATUS.

The Mouth and its appendages. Anatomy. The lingual cartilage. Worming. *Teeth,* their anatomy and physiology. TARTAR ACCUMULATIONS. BROKEN TEETH. EXCESSIVE WEAR. DISPLACEMENT. *Cutting and rasping the Tushes.* CARIES. ABSCESS OF THE JAW. "CANKER OF THE MOUTH." *Loss of Molars.* CLEFT PALATE. DISEASES OF THE TONGUE: GLOSSITIS. PARALYSIS. WOUNDS OF THE TONGUE, incised, punctured. BLAINE. Youatt's views. RANULA. *Ptyalism.* ULCERATION OF THE LIPS. WARTS IN THE MOUTH. PHARYNGITIS. Anatomy of the œsophagus, stomach, and bowels. Sinuses of Morgagni. *Diseases and accidents of the Œsophagus.* STRICTURE. *Filaria sanguinolenta.* CHOKING. *Œsophagotomy. Some general symptoms of disorder of the alimentary canal:* INAPPETENCE, INDIGESTION, Pyrosis, VOMITION, persistent vomition. COLIC. DIARRHŒA. CONSTIPATION, COSTIVENESS, and TORPIDITY OF THE BOWELS. DISEASES OF THE STOMACH: GASTRIC CATARRH, "Husk," GASTRITIS, ULCER OF THE STOMACH, GASTRIC FISTULA, GASTRIC DILATATION. FOREIGN BODIES IN THE STOMACH. Observations by Mr. W. Hunting. Youatt's cases. PARASITES: *Ascaris marginata, Spiroptera sanguinolenta, Olulanus tricuspis* (of the cat). Whether dogs should be allowed to feed on bones? DISEASES OF THE INTESTINES: ENTERITIS. Blaine on rheumatic enteritis. DYSENTERY, IMPACTION, *Calculus* rare, *Volvulus* not recorded. INVAGINATION or INTUSSUSCEPTION. Laparotomy. Mayhew's views on cæcal disease. PROLAPSUS RECTI *v.* ANI. HÆMORRHOIDS or PILES. *Fistula in Ano.* Atony of the Rectum. STRICTURE OF THE BOWEL: Mr. A. Broad's views. ABDOMINAL HERNIÆ rare in dog. EPIPLOCELE. *Femoral and Inguinal Herniæ :* Hill and Friederberger's cases. *Ventral Hernia.* WORMS IN THE BOWELS. "Maw worms." *Ascaris marginata.* Other round worms found in the intestines of the dog. Tapeworms. *Tænia cucumerina, T. cænurus, T. marginata, T. echinococcus, T. serrata, T. literata,* and *Bothriocephalus latus.* The corresponding cystic worms. Tæniafuges. *Holostoma* and *Cheiracanthus.* POLYPUS RECTI.

APPENDIX 1.—THE DISEASES AND SURGERY OF THE PERITONEUM AND BELLY: LAPAROTOMY, PERITONITIS, ASCITES. Differential diagnosis. "TAPPING THE BELLY" *v.* PARACENTESIS ABDOMINIS.

APPENDIX 2.—THE LIVER, PANCREAS, AND SPLEEN, &c.: Anatomy of the liver and gall-bladder. HEPATITIS, Acute. "Bilious inflammation of the bowels." Mayhew's case of liver abscess. Chronic. DEGENERATIONS OF THE LIVER, Rupture, MALIGNANT

xii   CONTENTS.

PAGE

DISEASE, PARASITIC DISEASE. *Distoma conjunctum*. Echinococci recorded by Reiman. *Filaria hepatica*, by Mather. *Ectopia hepatis*. The *Excretory Apparatus of the Liver*. BILIARY FISTULA. BILIARY CALCULI. *Pancreas:* its duct. Bernard's case of absorption of the pancreas. *Spleen*. SPLENITIS. Excision of the organ. HÆMORRHAGIC TUMOURS. Rupture of the spleen. Splenic apoplexy. Sarcomatous growth in, and other malignant disease of, the spleen. *Diseases of the other ductless glands:* Thyroid body. BRONCHOCELE or GOITRE ("Kernels"). Youatt on heredity in this disease, and his account of acute cases. The thymus body . . 98—152

CHAPTER VII.—THE URINARY APPARATUS.

Anatomy. *Diseases of the Kidneys*. ALBUMINOUS NEPHRITIS (Bright's disease). Accounts of the disorder by Axe and Mathis. NEPHRITIS *v*. RETINITIS. RENAL CALCULUS. Atrophy and hypertrophy of kidney. Hydatids (Blaine), more probably cysts of retention. *Parasites*. *Eustrongylus gigas*. Ureter blocked by calculus or dilated. CYSTITIS. Epizooty recorded by Blaine and Youatt. CYSTIC CALCULUS, induced artificially by Boerhaave. Mayhew on diagnosis of stone in the bladder. LITHOTOMY. Hill's case. Youatt's mention of natural lithotrity. RUPTURE OF THE BLADDER. CYSTIC HERNIA. Stricture of neck and eversion not recorded. ABNORMAL URINATION. Retention, Suppression, Scantiness, Strangury, Incontinence. PARALYSIS OF THE BLADDER. *Passing the Catheter*. Profuse staling. The urine of carnivora contrasted with that of herbivora. HÆMATURIA. DIABETES MELLITUS, by Prof. Ferraro. Urine with copious sediment. PROSTATIC DISEASE. Mannington and MacGillivray's cases. Frequence of this disorder. URETHRITIS, BALANITIS, and POSTHITIS. GONORRHŒA. Stricture and spasm of the urethra. Séon's case of parasite in the urethra. URETHRAL CALCULUS   .   .   .   .   .   153—164

CHAPTER VIII.—THE GENERATIVE APPARATUS.

OF THE MALE: Anatomy and physiology. Structure of the penis. Lauscat's description of its glans. The phenomenon of "locking" in sexual union. POSTHITIS. WARTY GROWTHS. "*Polypi of the Sheath*" (Blaine). *Congenital malformation of the Penis. Imperforate Prepuce*. AMPUTATION OF THE PENIS. INFLAMMATION OF THE SCROTUM. CASTRATION. IMPOTENCE. *Sarcocele*. ORCHITIS. Scirrhous Testis. OF THE FEMALE: OVARIOTOMY. *Atrophy*

PAGE

of the ovaries. Malignant disease. METRITIS: caused by artificial attempts to induce œstrum. *Ulceration of the lining Mucous Membrane.* Yeoman's case. HYDROMETRA or HYDROPS UTERI. UTERINE DISPLACEMENTS. HERNIA UTERI *v.* HYSTEROCELE. Rainard's case. Selle's case. Corby's case. Kopp's case. *Torsio uteri.* PROLAPSUS UTERI or "Inversion." Differential diagnosis. Restoration by taxis. AMPUTATIO UTERI, or *Excision of the Womb.* Leech's case. Broad's method. Brown's case complicated with *Uterine Tumour. Uterine inertia* (Fleming). POST-PARTUM HÆMORRHAGE. Mayhew's case. LACERATION OF THE VAGINAL WALLS. "*Cancer,*" or TUMOURS OF THE VAGINA. True CANCER. *Lipomata. Condylomata, "Warts." Fibromata. Polypus.* LEUCORRHŒA. *Inversio v.* PROLAPSUS VAGINÆ. Rainard's *method of amputation.* "*Infibulation.*" PASSAGE OF THE CATHETER. PARTURITION AND OTHER SPECIAL PHYSIOLOGICAL PHENOMENA OF THE FEMALE: *Œstrum.* SUPERFŒTATION. *Spurious Pregnancy* (Fleming's account). Absence of œstrum. Constant desire. PREGNANCY: *False pains.* Hygiene of pregnancy. PARTURITION: normal. Difficulty not common. Reasons for this. *Malposition of the Fœtus.* Assistance to be rendered at parturition. *Premature Birth and Abortion.* DELAYED PARTURITION. OPERATIVE INTERFERENCES: embryotomy. Cephalotomy. *Mayhew's Parturition instrument.* Extractors. Forceps. The crochet, as described by Mayhew. The new-born pup and fœtal membranes. Monstrous conditions. *Moles or anidian monsters.* EXTRA-UTERINE FŒTATION. CÆSAREAN OPERATIONS: Franck's statistics. Feser's cases. Adam's method of operation. *After-treatment of Parturient Animals.* Overstraining the milking powers. Adoption of a foster mother. Liability of bitch to eat her pups. The lochia.

APPENDIX.—ORGANS AND PROCESS OF LACTATION AND THEIR DISORDERS: The mammary glands and milk. RETENTION OF MILK. "Milk abscess," *and concretions in the ducts of the teats.* MAMMITIS. *Lacteal Fistula.* MALIGNANT GROWTHS OF THE MAMMARY GLAND. TUMOURS. To "dry up" a bitch. Warty growths and "chaps" of the teats . . . 165—198

CHAPTER IX.—THE NERVOUS SYSTEM.

Extreme nervousness of temperament of some breeds of dogs as a special feature in canine surgery and medicine. *Neuralgia.* Williams's views as to mental disorders. Epilepsy. *Vertigo.* Mégnin on epileptiform acariasis. Maybew's precautions for dealing with "fits." APOPLEXY, the *parturient form.* INJURIES TO THE HEAD Concussion, Compression, Fracture (Symond's case), Apoplectic complications. ENCEPHALITIS: Leblanc's case. Gowing's case. HYDROCEPHALUS: Illustrative case. Parasites. PARALYSIS. Blaine on *Acupuncturation*. Stross on spinal pachymeningitis. Locomotor ataxy. PUERPERAL ECLAMPSIA: Fleming's account of this disorder. CHOREA or St. Vitus's Dance. Gowers and Sankey on its pathological anatomy. Harley's artificial production of the disease. CRAMP. TETANUS. *Opisthotonos and Pleurosthotonos*. Coats on the pathology of the disorder . . . 199—213

CHAPTER X.—THE ORGANS OF SPECIAL SENSE.

THE EYE: Anatomical comparison with that of horse. ULCERATION OF THE EYELIDS: "*Watery Eye*," entropion, ectropium, trichiasis. *Obstruction of the Lachrymal Duct. Laceration of the Supra-orbital Ligament*. TUMOURS ON CARTILAGO NICTITANS. CONJUNCTIVITIS and SIMPLE OPHTHALMIA. Granular conjunctivitis. ULCERATION OF THE CORNEA. STAPHYLOMA. Opacity. DROPSY OF THE AQUEOUS CHAMBER. Traumatic distension of the eyeball. DERMOID TUMOURS. CATARACT. Accidental extraction of the lens by a cat. AMAUROSIS. DISLOCATION OF THE EYEBALL. *Extirpation of the Eyeball*. Persistence of Membrana pupillaris (Youatt). Inflammation of the iris and choroid. THE EAR: Ear-ache. *Otitis*. Deafness, peculiar form resulting from too low " cropping." INTERNAL CANKER, Coculet's treatment. EXTERNAL CANKER. *Amputation of Dogs' Ears* (" cropping" or " rounding "). Ear caps (Peuch's, Hill's, Mayhew's). TICKS IN THE EAR. Scurfiness of the flap. HÆMATOMA or SERO-SANGUINEOUS ABSCESS OF THE FLAP: Hunting's, Mayhew's, and Trinchera's method of treatment. AURICULAR ACARIASIS: accounts by Mégnin and Nocard. *Polypi of the Ear*. THE SKIN: Empirical notions on the subject. Views of various canine pathologists. Anatomy of the skin of the dog. *Foulness*. SIMPLE ERYTHEMA. ECZEMA (*True dermatitis* or "*Surfeit*"). Pityriasis and psoriasis. Gamgee on mercurial eczema. *Pruritus. Alopecia* or "*Baldness*." VERRUCÆ or "*Warts*." ANASARCA. Erysipelas (?). PARASITIC AFFECTIONS. DERMATOZOA: General remarks on the diseases to which they give rise. TRUE MANGE or SARCOPTIC SCABIES. Detection of sarcoptes and symbiotes. " Dry," " scabby," and " watery" mange. " Red mange." Special points concerning the treatment of parasitic skin diseases. Blaine on mange dressings. The preparations suggested by different canine pathologists. FOLLICULAR MANGE. The characters of *Demodex folliculorum*. Gruby's experiments with it. Hunting on treatment of the disease. Various authors on this subject. *Skin*

PAGE

disease due to Leptus autumnalis, the Harvest Bug, described by Friedberger and Fleming. TICKS: Anderssen on the husk tick of South Africa. FLEAS: various methods for removal of them. LICE. THE DERMATOPHYTIC DISEASES OF THE DOG: their general characters. St. Cyr's conclusions. TINEA TONSURANS *v.* "RINGWORM." Not to be confounded with *Simple Herpes.* TINEA FAVOSA *v.* "HONEYCOMB RINGWORM." . . . 214—244

CHAPTER XI.—THE LOCOMOTOR SYSTEM.

Separation of Epiphyses. FRACTURE: of walls of cranium, of lower jaw, of vertebræ, of ribs, of pelvis, of bones of the fore limb. Treatment of fractures. Blaine on application of splints. Peuch on fractured tibia. Mayhew on setting fractures. Fractured metatarsals. *False Joint.* DISLOCATIONS: of elbow-joint, of shoulder, of knee, hock, patella, coxæ, femoral-joint, small joints of the foot. Luxation of the lower jaw. ANCHYLOSIS AND EXOSTOSIS. Stiff joints, splints, spavins. SPRAINS. Laceration of the trapezius muscle in the cat. The FOOT: examination of it as to soundness. *Sore or over-worn Feet.* "*Founder.*" Mange as affecting the feet. *Sinuous ulcer beneath the Claw.* Thorns. Wounds. *Overgrown Claws.* AMPUTATION OF THE TOE. "*Dew Claws.*" *Parasites between the Toes.* CONGENITAL DEFORMITIES OF THE LIMBS. Wolstenholme's case. *Tenotomy. Cancerous diseases of Bones, Ostitis, and Periostitis.* Amputation of the whole limb . . 245—257

CHAPTER XII.—POISONING.

In its practical aspects. Toxicological and other experiments with drugs on dogs. Idiosyncracies of these animals. CARBOLIC ACID, its specific action on carnivora. Broad, of Bath, his method of using it with safety, and his treatment for carbolic poisoning. Kunde's treatment in the same emergency. *Tobacco Water and Hellebore solutions.* MERCURY COMPOUNDS. Eczema mercuriale. Bennett on the effects of mercury on bones and its analogy to supposed syphilitic lesions. VEGETABLE POISONING. Not common in dog. How he obtains mineral poisons. *Treatment.* STRYCHNIA. Valenti on monobromide of camphor. Feser on the toxic action of strychnia nitrate. Butler's successful case of strychnia poisoning. *Lead poisoning.* EUTHANASIA. Carbonic-acid poisoning (Dr.

Richardson). Electric shock. Drowning. *Prussic Acid*. SNAKE
BITE. *Curara poison*. Not to be used in vivisection. Stings of
venomous insects . . . . 258—264

CHAPTER XIII.—MINOR SURGERY.

TUMOURS: *Malignant*. Frequent in dog. Care essential when using
chloroform for operations. *Melanosis. Sarcomata.* NON-MALIG-
NANT, *Fibrous or Fibro-vascular growths, Simple fibroma, Fibro-
cystic Tumours.* "Capped hock" and "Capped elbow." *Warty
growths. Fatty and Osseous Tumours.* WOUNDS: their general
nature, causes, and peculiarities in dogs. Reference to Parkes'
experiments on gunshot wounds of the abdomen. Fleming on the
best method of separating and securing fighting dogs . 265—268

TABULAR STATEMENT OF MEDICINES FOR INTERNAL AND EXTERNAL
USE . . . . . . 269—277

LIST OF ILLUSTRATIONS.

FIG.   PAGE

1. Physiognomy of disease in dogs as depicted by Mayhew—Pneumonia   9
2.   ,,   ,,   ,,   ,,   Asthma   .   9
3.   ,,   ,,   ,,   ,,   Gastritis .   9
4.   ,,   ,,   ,,   ,,   Colic   .   9
5.   ,,   ,,   ,,   ,,   Rheumatism   9
6, 7. Administration of medicines—pills (Mayhew) . . . 15
8.   ,,   ,,   liquid (Mayhew) . . . 16
9. Dog seton needle (Peuch and Toussaint) 22
10. Bandages for ears and abdomen (Peuch and Toussaint) . . 24
11. Method of fastening tape on a dog's nose to muzzle him (Mayhew) 25
12. Figure of mad dog (furious stage). After Sanson . . . 29
13.   ,,   ,,   (dumb form). After Sanson . . . 32
14. Pince collier pour saisir le chien (Peuch and Toussaint) . . 39
15. Bouley's sticks and rope for seizing suspicious dogs . . 39
16. Wire muzzle (after Fleming) 46
17. Bourrel's rasp and gag for teeth (Peuch and Toussaint) . . 47
18—21. Distemper organisms (after Kreijewski) . . . 49
22. Surra organisms, spirilloids 58
23. Rachitic dog (Hill) 67
24. General representation of circulatory organs of the dog (Chauveau) 74
25. Fatty degeneration (Quain) 75
26. Fatty infiltration (Quain) 75
27. Pentastome (Cobbold) . . , . . . 85
28, 29. Parasites of verminous bronchitis (from Hill on ' Dogs,' after Osler) 93
30. Arnold's patent syringe for intratracheal injection . . . 97
31. Arnold's improved patent hypodermic syringe . . . 97
32 and 33. Dog's teeth (Chauveau). Anterior and lateral views . 99
34. Intestines and omentum major (after Chauveau) . . . 109
35. Throat forceps (Arnold) 110
36. Stomach (after Chauveau) 118
37—39. Parasites (after Stonehenge) 134, 135
40. Liver, &c. (from Fleming's translation of Chauveau's ' Anatomy ') . 140
41. Liver disorder (Mayhew) 144
42. Distoma conjunctum (after Cobbold) 146

b

LIST OF ILLUSTRATIONS.

FIG.	PAGE
43. Pancreas (after Gamgee)	148
44. Eustrongylus gigas (after Cobbold)	155
45, 46. Cystic calculi (after Morton)	157
47. Os penis (after Strangeways, by Vaughan)	165
48. Gravid uterus of a multiparous mammal contrasted with that of the human female (from Fleming's 'Obstetrics')	182
49. Mayhew's parturition instrument	188
50. Mayhew's crochet	189
51—56. Forceps and extractors of various kinds (after Fleming)	190, 191
57. Fœtus in its membranes (Fleming)	192
58—61. Aspects of cerebral hemispheres of cat, life-size	202
62—65. „ „ of dog (retriever), life-size	203
66—68. Ear-caps—66 (Peuch and Toussaint), 67 (Mayhew), 68 (Hill)	222, 223
69. Sarcoptes canis (Gerlach)	231
70, 71. Parasites in skin-follicles of dog, follicular scabies (Williams, after Gruby)	235
72. Acari folliculorum in hair-follicles, and also in sebaceous glands (Gruby)	236
73. Leptus autumnalis (Friedberger)	239
74. Achorion Lebertii (after Fleming)	242
75, 76. Achorion Schönleinii, illustrating stages of development (Bennett)	243
77. Thalli, mycelia, and sporidia of Achorion (Bennett)	244
78. Tinea favosa crusts in various stages (Bennett)	244
79. Skeleton of the dog (Chauveau)	247
80. Method of setting fractured legs (Mayhew)	249
81. Bandage for fractured scapula (Hill)	251
82. Dislocation of shoulder-joint (Hill)	251
83. Muscles of forearm and foot of the dog (Chauveau)	253
84. Muscles of antero-external aspect of forearm and foot (Chauveau)	255
85. Bones of forearm and foot of dog (Chauveau)	255
86. Skeleton of dog illustrating the effects of mercury (Bennett)	260
87, 88. Two views of the femur of the same (Bennett)	261

THE

DISEASES OF THE DOG.

CHAPTER I.—INTRODUCTION—GENERAL REMARKS.

A WORK on the dog has an all but universal interest. It is almost impossible to enumerate in full the various sporting uses to which this noble and sagacious animal has been put: greyhound, foxhound, beagle, and their allies; pointer, retriever, setter, spaniel; terriers of various kinds and most mongrels are all more or less used in *sport*, and all by their conformation and mental qualities have been adapted to their special duties through the long-continued and skilled regulation of their breeding operations by intelligent men. In *war* the use of dogs is reviving; recently an organised dog service for sentry duty at outposts has been officially originated in Russia; and it certainly seems a legitimate method of defence in those wars where the acute senses and stealthy movements of the savage are apt to be pitted against senses blunted by civilisation and movements cramped by discipline. The fierce bloodhound tracking the runaway negro slave through marsh and over mountain may not be pleasing to our minds, but when we see his instincts turned to the detection of murderers and other criminals we agree that they are being put to a legitimate use. In *agriculture* throughout the world the dog finds scope for honorable and useful work, whether in the care of sheep, in the extermination of predatory rodents, or the defence of farm buildings. In *travel*, whether in search of the Poles or "Through the Dark Continent," the dog is a necessary part of the bold explorer's equipment. In *trade* some use is made of the dog in the defence of property; but his qualities are not mercantile, he is adapted neither for pack nor cart, and although attempts have been made to force him to settle down to the quiet ways of trade in the service of the cats'-meat man, happily the law has stepped in to prevent such a perversion of the uses to which the dog was intended by nature. Arctic explorers, indeed, above the highest latitude of the reindeer, legitimately use teams of dogs of the grand Esquimaux breed, but serious mortality from epizootic diseases is a sad drawback to such use, and threatens the poor Esquimaux with practical loss of his best friend. The *humane operations* of the dogs of St. Bernard are well known.

We have hitherto represented our canine companion as an essentially feudal animal, and so he remains to the end; prompt in attack, sudden in raid, fierce in onslaught, obstinate and relentless in pursuit, skilled in the driving and protection of flocks, watchful on guard, and, withal, of an adventuresome and exploring turn of mind—when not more seriously engaged bringing all his valuable faculties keenly to bear on the chase—that "mimicry of noble war;" altogether he much reminds us of a Border forayer such as Scott loved to portray.

Although thus bold in the field he is also a very accomplished "Carpet Knight;" his eyes beaming with intelligence and trustful love, his docile temper, his lively temperament, all his points and qualities adapt him as the trusted and loved companion of woman and the friend of man. He has often become strangely changed in consequence into the so-called "fancy" breeds. To fit him for the boudoir and the dwelling-house man has so artificially selected him that some dogs have no hair and others are completely concealed by their more or less beautiful locks; some dogs are light of limb as the most delicate deer, others resemble a prize-fighter in build; some have their faces so shortened that there is no room for the full complement of teeth granted by nature, and some all but entirely refuse their natural flesh food and become as pampered and fastidious in their diet as human epicures.

But man's interference with the works of nature has not been without its drawbacks. As the varieties of the dog are so numerous and his uses so varied, we find that his diseases and accidents are very important and diversified. Whereas the hunting dog generally suffers little from disease and much from accidents to which his reiving habits expose him, and spends his life in a state of hard "condition," at the other extreme we find the ladies' lap-dog, whose stomach refuses all but the most delicate morsels artificially prepared, whose limbs can scarcely support his weight, whose natural atmosphere is that of a close and heated room, and who has become petulant and snappish through the enervating influence of his surroundings. It is commonly said that so diverse are the manners of dogs of the sporting and fancy breeds, that he who is competent to treat the diseases of the one is not best adapted to deal with those of the other. This is not correct. The science and practice of canine pathology is applicable to all dogs—for "a dog is a dog all the world over." The skilful practitioner duly considers all the special features of each case, both in the determination of the nature of an attack and in the adoption of proper remedial measures. He certainly has a very difficult task, for in no branch of medical practice are the cases more obscure, the action and doses of medicines more complicated, and the niceties of treatment more elaborate than in canine surgery and medicine.

It may well be asked whether the practitioner of human medicine or of veterinary surgery is the more competent to treat the dog when diseased. On the one hand, it may be urged that the dog is now practically an omnivore; he lives in such close association with man that he is affected by like disease-producing influences and is exposed to the same contingencies of life. On the other, that the education and practice of the veterinarian is the more universal and varied, and that he is specially instructed in the details of disease, anatomy, physiology, and therapeutics of the dog. The latter considerations must bear the most weight, but we must not lose sight of the fact that in the present day veterinary science is becoming so complex that during the period of time devoted by students to it but little attention can be given to the details of canine science, which needs, however, much care and time for appreciation of its specialities. Thus few veterinarians are really good canine pathologists, indeed it is only in London and some of our other large cities, where competition is keen and valuable dogs are numerous, that a veterinary practitioner can afford to consider dog practice on a par with that of horses and cattle. Any veterinary student at college can obtain a good practical and a fair theoretical acquaintance with the diseases of the dog; only a few graduates can afford to develop this knowledge into a speciality of practice. These remarks are made with a view to thoroughly establishing the position that to be a veterinary practitioner is not necessarily to be a canine practitioner; the two classes of practice, although generally combined, are really quite distinct. At the same time the veterinary surgeon is by education and practice best adapted in all cases to treat diseases of the dog. YOUATT and BLAINE in the past and GOWING of Camden Town in the present, are notable instances of veterinary surgeons who were (or are) also accomplished canine pathologists; and if asked to enumerate some London canine pathologists of the present time we may reply Gowing of Camden Town; Rowe of Regent's Park; Hunting of Down Street, Piccadilly; and Sewell. We name them in no spirit of advertisement, nor as implying that they are not also skilled veterinary surgeons, but simply with a view to giving honour where honour is due we mention them as specialists in canine pathology, who are assisting to lay the foundation of an enormous development of this branch of medical science.

Mr. HUNTING started some little time ago a course of special instruction in canine pathology, but the movement was in advance of the times, and, we believe, was, after the first course, discontinued. There can be no doubt that before long the public will be sufficiently impressed with a movement of this kind to give it adequate support.

Few branches of medical practice are more beset with empirics than this. We are constantly hearing of men who are "good hands with dogs," who certainly have attained a fair amount of skill in minor operations and nursing, and so are better than the absolutely ignorant, but who are not to be trusted in the treatment of disease, for they have a knowledge neither of the interior economy of the dog nor of the action of the medicines which they use. They like medicines which show some clear and indubitable evidence of their action, hence the very frequent and excessive use commonly made of emetics and cathartics in canine practice.

There is a delicacy of manipulation and a refinement in practice needed in the medical treatment of dogs which is not required so much in the treatment of larger animals. The tissues are very delicate, the nervous organisation is high, these patients can be more readily handled and controlled than the larger forms, and are generally nursed and tended with greater assiduity. Much tact, too, is needed in management of dog owners, especially where the fancy breeds are concerned. The pain necessarily inflicted at times for the ultimate benefit of the patient proves distressing to the fair owner; instructions as to strict regimen are liable to be infringed through mistaken kindness; and there are a number of other disturbing elements in most dog cases with which the medical adviser soon becomes familiar.

The dog, as a carnivorous mammal, differs from the herbivora in a number of essential and important respects. That his movements may be prompt, free, and swift, his *skeleton* is light, and its component parts dense to atone for want of bulk; they are also numerous, and have well-developed processes for the attachment of muscles. There is not nearly so much fibrous tissue in the carnivora as the herbivora, the muscles of the former being adapted rather for sharp powerful action than for sustained and slow exertion. We find (for instance) none of those remarkable fibrous arrangements by which the horse is enabled to sleep standing and to thoroughly rest himself without lying down. The *digestive apparatus* is relatively much less bulky, especially the dental and intestinal portions. The molar teeth being small and short-fanged the skull requires neither large sinuses nor bulky jaws, hence it is light, and only a very small ligamentum nuchæ is required, with which again is associated the absence of long anterior dorsal spines, such as constitute "withers." The flesh food is easily digestible, and so the main operations of the process are carried on in the stomach, which is large, while the bowels are short, straight, and small; consequently the total bulk of abdominal contents is small, and so the belly has but little superficial abdominal fascia to support its viscera. Vigorous and active movements entail a well-developed *nervous and circulatory system,* and from this result also well-developed kidneys, liver, and lungs; the latter being associated with wide air-passages, and a remarkably elastic and capacious chest, which narrows anteriorly to allow free play to the *fore limbs*. These latter are somewhat prehensile as well as adapted for locomotive purposes. Thus, there is a small clavicle, the ulna is very well developed and freely rotatory on the radius, and there are five digits armed with claws and each more or less endowed with special muscles. In the *hind limb* the arrangements are on very much the same pattern, but the power of rotation is much more limited, and one digit is atrophied and thrown out of work. All the *organs of sense* are well developed, as being much required to enable the animal in a state of nature to procure its food, also the emergencies of its life sharpen its faculties, increase its intelligence, and enlarge its *brain*. As the young are born in a very helpless state and are naturally subjected to many emergencies and vicissitudes dogs are polyparous, the number at a birth varying much. When nature's means of preventing dogs becoming over-numerous (such as the influences of starvation and the predations of more powerful carnivora) are partially or wholly inoperative the effects are very serious. This is seen to an extent in some Eastern cities in the present day, where dogs go about in bands and prove a great nuisance; also the early Australian colonists had to wage fierce war against the dogs, who bred freely and preyed upon flocks of sheep.

Liability to disease is directly influenced by the size and functional activity of organs, semi-wild dogs are not predisposed to any special diseases, but artificial selection materially alters the state of affairs. It disturbes the wholesome balance which has been by nature established between the organs and systems of organs, and those parts which become especially developed are thereby predisposed to disease. The deleterious effects of domestication are very well marked in the prevalence of nervous disorder and cancer among fancy breeds, of rheumatism among sporting dogs, and of canker of the ear and mange among long-haired and long-eared animals. Almost all the disorders of dogs thus arise from man's mismanagement and tampering with natural conditions. Disease is not a necessary attendant on variation, but the latter must be considered a most important predisposing cause.

We must accept as established by observation the following statements:—That carnivora among mammals have, as such, some special features of disease; dogs among carnivores, different breeds among dogs, and individual dogs among those of a breed; or, in other words, order, genus, species, variety, and individual, influence the type and character of disease.

Want of care in regulation of surrounding influences is a fruitful cause of disease; by *gradual* change the constitution may become adapted to the most varied conditions of diet, climate, and work, but *sudden* transitions throw the animal economy into disorder. Thus the dog has almost become a herbivore in some cases, and indeed generally is an omnivore; so greatly has the influence of changed diet affected the system that the very teeth are altered accordingly; but if we suddenly change any dog from a flesh diet to meal food disease will result. Again, with regard to climate, no animal has become more universally diffused than the dog, and he has become adapted by variation to the climate of each country, but ordinary English breeds if imported into India rapidly succumb to the exhausting effects of sudden change of climate, unless they be taken very great care of. Finally, although largely due to the effects of breeding, the marked difference between the greyhound and the bulldog is also a result of their special work, and neither could be put to the work of the other without serious ill-consequences. Age, sex, and various physiological conditions, such as those of lactation and pregnancy, are, in dogs as in other animals, active *predisposing causes* of disease. The *exciting causes* in general are too numerous to be mentioned in detail here.

The GENERAL SYMPTOMS OF DISEASE in the dog are, in the main, departure from ordinary habits, such as dulness, want of appetite, an unthrifty appearance, the animal being unsocial and endeavouring to hide himself,—they consist in those slight divergences from ordinary habits which will best be recognised by the master; soon more marked signs of disorder set in and enable us to diagnose the case.* Fever is an accompaniment of most diseases and is easily recognisable ; we shall treat of it in detail hereafter. Although the arterial system of the dog is well developed, the *pulse* is not so good and reliable a guide as it is in diseases of the horse or man. Many dogs are very nervous, and it will be found that when they are handled by a stranger the pulse runs up so rapidly as to render it anything but a reliable guide. It should always be taken, however, and with as much gentleness as possible. The character of the beat gives us some information, and the knowledge thus acquired increases with experience. The number can best be taken at the heart by placing the

* Mayhew lays great stress on the physiognomy of disease in dogs, and rightly so. Although his illustrations (as appended) are exaggerated they have a certain value in fixing on the memory the position assumed in various disorders.

INTRODUCTION. 9

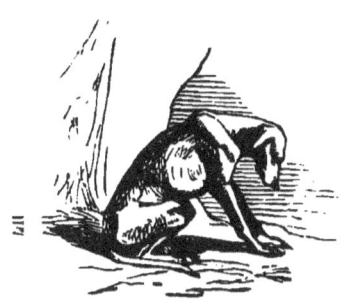

Fig. 1.—Inflammation of lungs.

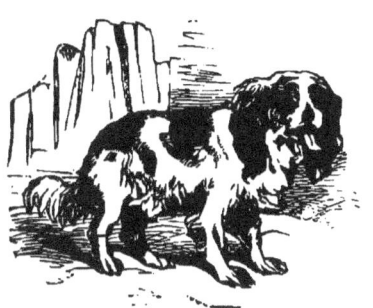

Fig. 2.—Asthma.

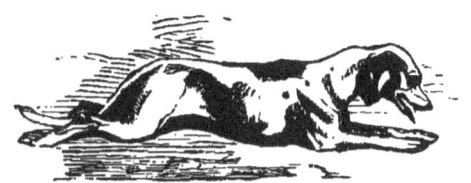

Fig. 3.—Gastritis.

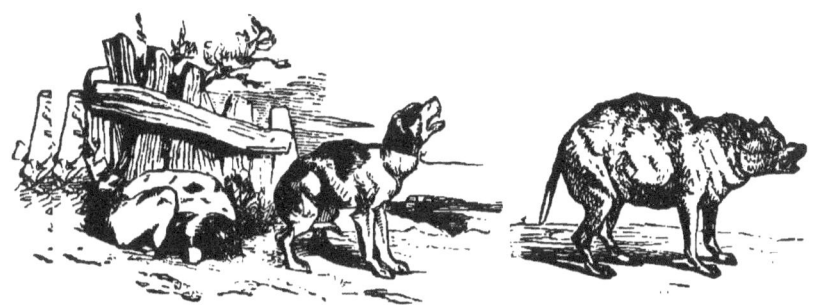

Fig. 4.—Colic.   Fig. 5.—Rheumatism.

(The physiognomy of disease in dogs, as depicted by MAYHEW.)

hands firmly one against each side; the heart-sounds are distinct on auscultation. The character of the beats can be determined either above the wrist (as is usual in human practice), or inside the elbow, or from the femoral artery inside the thigh. The normal beat of the dog's pulse averages 100—120 per minute, but the character as well as number of the beats varies much with the breed.*

The *respirations* can best be taken by auscultation or by observation of the movements of the nostril, but they vary so much in health as to afford us really very little guidance. The colour of the *mucous membranes* gives us the best indications of the state of the circulation; the state of the skin and nose, also the temperature of the limbs, assist us in our diagnosis. Auscultation is our main guide in testing the respirations and heart's beat. Also we can learn much from the *general behaviour of the animal* and *the state of his ejecta* is of value in informing us as to the nature of his diseases.

The *internal temperature* has only recently been recognised as a valuable guide in canine diagnosis and prognosis; the thermometer may be inserted inside the cheek, or in the anus, or vulva. The range in normal internal temperature of the dog is 100°—104° F.

PROGNOSIS is generally favorable; it is really wonderful what serious injuries dogs will undergo without fatal effects, and disease makes serious ravages before death ensues, but we must always remember the liability of dogs to sudden death from convulsions.

TREATMENT of dogs is a very delicate matter; the doses to be given are small and require careful adjustment, often frequent repetition. In canine more than veterinary practice "placebos" are required; the whims and humours of the dog and owner must often be tolerated, and inert agents administered, lest the owner think nothing is being done and be tempted to interfere with the case. There is much scope for zeal and energy of the nurse in superintending the numerous details of care of the sick animal.

* "When a dog pants violently his circulation may be considered as quickened" (Blaine).

In canine almost as much as in human practice must allowance be made for nervous influences. To those accustomed to handle only our domesticated herbivora under disease it will be somewhat difficult to recognise that sometimes in canine patients the nervous irritability constitutes the most serious feature of the attack. Chloral, opium, and ether are recognised as assuming a high place in the catalogue of dog medicines, and such nerve tonics as nitrate of silver and strychnia, also coffee and tea, are useful in the hands of the skilful canine physician. It is to ladies' pets, drawing-, and bed-room dogs, in fact, that these remarks especially apply—they are extremely tender under disease and suffer from intense mental feeling, and are particularly liable to chorea, fits, paralysis, and other nervous phenomena. It has been remarked, too, that in them delirium usually precedes death. Among such animals we sometimes find *" malingerers "*; strange as it may seem, it is an indubitable fact, amply established by experience, that many dogs at times feign sickness deliberately, perhaps with somewhat the same instinct as leads the fox, when hard pressed, to " sham " death. Again, it is such artificially bred and reared animals which, like spoilt children, require the greatest *tact and gentleness with firmness* on the part of the physician or surgeon in handling them for various purposes. They are apt to prove refractory, especially in the presence of their fair owners, who are too apt to support them in their mutiny against medical authority. There are a number of small details as to the handling of strange and refractory dogs which are to be learned in the school of experience. We must here insist that boldness is essential, freedom from roughness and the infliction of unnecessary pain must be adopted, and seclusion during the examination of the patient. The nervousness of dogs renders attention to the details of nursing very essential in canine practice. Fortunately, as a rule dogs have kind friends and caretakers, who will willingly do what they can to lessen the pain and discomfort of sickness, and are only apt to err on the side of " doing too much."

The DETAILS OF NURSING consist in strict attention to the animal's comfort and well-being in such matters as food, air, bedding, and administration or application of medicaments ; *warmth* is of much benefit to sick dogs, for it is found that convulsions are apt to result from exposure of them to cold ; extreme *quietude* and unobtrusiveness in treatment, regular administration, as gently as possible, of remedies in exact accordance with instructions ; strict *cleanliness* of the patient and his surroundings, comfortable arrangement of his bed, and free supply of *pure air* are details to be attended to in nursing. The *diet* must be tempting and thoroughly clean, but little weaknesses of the patient, as for pork or horse-flesh, should not be yielded to, nor the animal allowed to eat to excess. Some articles of diet are too stimulating to the skin and bowels to be admissible as food for sick animals. Food, except when used as a vehicle for medicines, should never be forced on a patient. A suitable diet (generally of boiled rice flavoured with a little soup, gravy, beef tea, or chicken broth) should be placed before the animal frequently, but if refused taken away and rejected, fresh food being placed before him the next time. Some forms of dog food may with advantage be used semi-medicinally, thus greaves or boiled cabbage mixed with soup causes a looseness of the bowels, and unboiled liver is valuable for a similar purpose, and will be taken when the vegetable matters are persistently refused. Boiled liver is of less value, but useful. In dogs used for outdoor work horse-flesh is valuable for conditioning, but except when much work is done it produces irritation of the skin and foul smell of the body, and is, therefore, described as "heating"; oatmeal has a similar effect. Certain articles of dog diet are commonly spoken of as "causing worms" or "producing mange," terms which require a little explanation ; tapeworm is certainly more liable to result from a flesh than from a vegetable diet, but will not be generated by the former if care be taken to ensure the absence from the meat of cystic larvæ of tæniæ, such as echinococci in the liver, slender-necked hydatids appended to the abdominal viscera, or measles in the flesh. No food can produce true mange, but stimulating articles of diet can produce the rashes and congestions of the skin commonly known as surfeits. Sick dogs seldom require *washing* entirely, as do healthy dogs occasionally, but the patient may be much refreshened by careful cleaning of the natural orifices with tepid water and by such slight grooming, in the form of combing and brushing out the coat, as suffices to prevent matting of the hair and the skin becoming foul. The amount of attention to the skin must be carefully regulated according to the case. *Exercise*, with care not to weary the animal, should be given in the fresh air whenever the case admits of it. Mayhew's remarks on the EXAMINATION OF DOG PATIENTS are very much to the point : " Petted dogs are best examined away from their homes and in the absence of anyone who has been in the habit of caressing them. . . . I usually carry such dogs into a room by myself, and commence by quickly but gently lifting them off their legs and throwing them upon their backs. This appears to take the creatures by surprise, and a little assurance soon allays any fear which the action may have excited. The dog seldom after resists, but permits itself to be freely handled. Should, however, any disposition to bite be exhibited, the hand ought immediately to grasp the throat, nor should the hold be relinquished until the creature is fully convinced of the inutility of its malice, and thoroughly assured that no injury is intended towards it. A few kind words, and the absence of anything approaching to severity, will generally accomplish the latter object in a short period."

The *relations of diseases of the dog to those of other animals, especially man,* is a matter of importance upon which we shall have sometimes to lay great stress ; in reference to rabies and parasitic diseases this branch of our inquiry attains its greatest importance.

CHAPTER II.—CANINE PHARMACY, MATERIA MEDICA, AND THERAPEUTICS.

BEARING in mind the nature and peculiarities of our canine patients, as above indicated, we must consider the *specialities of canine pharmacy*. Many tasteless pills of various sorts are to be purchased from the veterinary pharmaceutical chemists in London and other large towns, and they will be found neat, clean, cheap, and convenient for every-day routine practice, but they cannot be relied on to meet all requirements. As *excipients*, *diluents*, and *placebos* the syrups have some value, as that of poppies, of buckthorn, and of squills, in addition to their more active medicinal effects. Honey, too, more frequently finds a place in canine than in veterinary practice. Medicines, pleasantly flavoured, can be given as *electuaries*, placed on the animal's tongue for him to suck in, but generally for dogs the pill, draught, or enema is advocated.

PILLS may be given much larger than those generally used, but the small ones give least trouble; it is better, however, to give one large pill than several small ones. The following details require consideration in the administration of pills. *Firstly*, the size of the animal. When it is small it must be taken on the lap, when of medium size placed standing on its hind legs with, in both cases, its back to the operator. If the animal be very large the operator must stand with it between his legs. *Secondly*, some animals fight and scratch with the fore paws; their limbs must be held by an assistant or a cloth tightly tied so as to bind them to the chest. *Thirdly*, the jaws must be separated and kept apart. This is generally done by placing one hand so that the palm rests on the upper part of the muzzle, and pressing, with the fingers on one side and the thumb on the other, the soft parts of the cheeks between the molar teeth; every effort to bite then pains the animal itself (Fig. 6). Sometimes it is necessary to draw the jaws of very large dogs apart by tape tied one piece round each jaw behind the tusks and drawing them

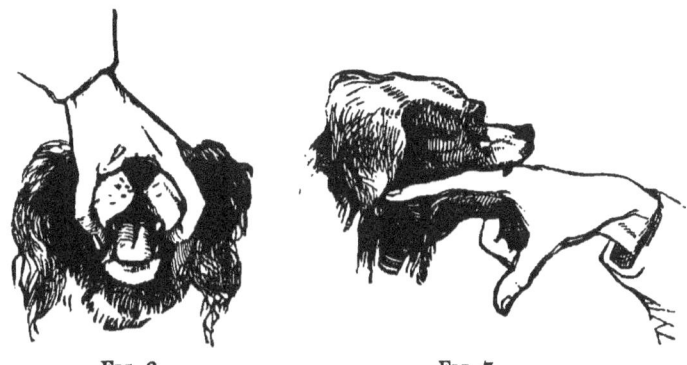

FIG. 6.   FIG. 7.

Administration of medicines. (MAYHEW.)

forcibly apart, but the head must at the same time be supported firmly from behind, in order that it may not be drawn away. *Fourthly,* with the unoccupied hand the pill must be placed well in the isthmus of the fauces, on the back of the tongue, and generally it is an advantage to give it a forcible impetus backwards by pressure from the index finger (Fig. 7). In a little while, the animal having been at once released but his mouth kept shut, he will (on being allowed to open the mouth again) begin to lick his nose, and, if not very sick, to wag his tail, evidently well pleased with himself.

This method of administration presents difficulties only in the case of large, strong dogs and to them, if not "off their feed," it is better to administer tasteless substances placed in the centre of a piece of meat which will be promptly bolted. Even substances with some strong taste or odour may be given in this way, but it should never be adopted in the case of animals with doubtful appetite, as they may discover or suspect the deceit and go altogether off their feed. Some substances of a pleasant taste or smell can be given in food or water, a very useful method in cases which require a long course of alterative or other treatment. To prevent expulsion of medicines by vomition, the head may be kept elevated for half an hour after administration.

DRAUGHTS should seldom exceed a wineglassful in bulk, generally a dessert-spoonful as a dose will suffice. They may be given with a spoon or from the phial itself. The dog being placed as above directed for giving a pill, the third act consists in drawing out the loose, soft part of the cheek so that it may form a sort of funnel when the head is elevated (Fig. 8). The head should be held up by an assistant. One hand of the administerer is used for pulling out the cheek and the other for pouring in the liquid gradually to replace that which trickles between the molars and down the animal's throat to be swallowed in successive gulps. A very small amount of liquid may be given by simply pouring it from a teaspoon on to the back

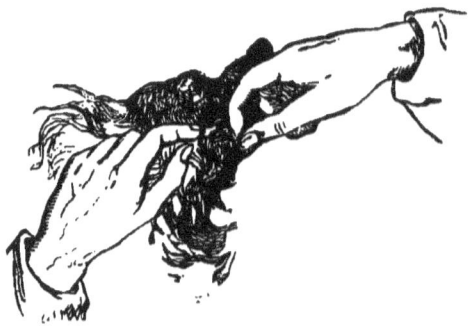

FIG. 8.—Administration of medicines. (MAYHEW.)

of the tongue, the mouth being held open as though for giving a pill. Coughing or attempts to cough should cause immediate cessation of the drenching process, but there is less liability to entry of fluid into the air-passages of the dog than of the horse, because the epiglottis of the former animal is relatively much the broader. In cases of emergency, fluid medicines may be administered by means of the *stomach pump*, or *subcutaneous injection syringe* ; but, with regard to the latter means, especially, we must remember that in some cases, and with some patients, even the slight necessary puncture might bring on convulsions.

ENEMATA for the dog must be small in bulk because his large intestine is not capacious. They are a very useful means of administration of medicine and nourishment. When judiciously resorted to they may be made to add very much to the comfort of a sick animal by preventing irritant accumulations in the bowel, such as are apt to give rise to colic or convulsions. They prove also directly useful *for removal of worms* when any occur in the large bowel. With some valuable dogs enemata may be required periodically as *a matter of kennel routine*, and it must be remembered that, almost always, enemata are a safer and simpler means of *arousing torpid bowels* than doses of purgative medicine. A syringe capable of containing from four ounces to a pint should be used according to the size of the dog. If the fluid is to be retained as *nutriment* or medicine, it should be small in quantity and of a bland, mucilaginous character. In all cases the nozzle of the syringe should be introduced very carefully and previously well lubricated. In cases of constipation it is always advisable to explore with the oiled forefinger beforehand in order to determine whether there is a large, dry, hard mass of fæces to be broken down. As an ordinary laxative means, warm water with some soap rubbed up in it is the best enema. Mucilage of starch, linseed tea, gruel, broth, milk, and so on, are given as nutritives in the form of enema, in doses of about one pint. When prompt catharsis is to be induced by enema, castor oil, oil of turpentine, and common salt, of each half an ounce, may be given with about eight ounces of gruel. As an *anodyne enema*, useful in certain forms of colic, laudanum, sulphuric ether, and spirits of turpentine, of each one to two drachms, may be given similarly.

CANINE MATERIA MEDICA differs in several very important respects from that of ordinary veterinary practice. Thus emetics assume a prominent place ; a quantity of pleasantly tasting substances, such as the syrups, must be added to the list of excipients; expectorants and vermifuges are of much importance. Again the question of doses is one which requires careful study and is not to be based on any consideration of the relative sizes of the horse and dog. There are certain special features about the action of some drugs which we shall require to remember.

CATHARTICS.—It is really extraordinary the differences of opinion of various authors about the action of remedies on the dog. The explanation lies in the very great differences in size and habits of the different varieties, so that the town and country canine practitioners arrive at very conflicting conclusions. Thus Prof. Dick prefers jalap one drachm, or an ounce of syrup of buckthorn, to aloes, which he considers uncertain, whereas Blaine and Youatt consider aloes in doses from a quarter to one drachm " the best and safest aperient for the dog." Mayhew says aloes is *not* a purgative to the dog. We may accept the following conclusions concerning cathartics as fairly correct :—

Aloes may be given in very large doses and is uncertain in its action on the dog. It is not a good cathartic for this animal, nor to be relied upon in the treatment of disease. *Jalap*, in doses of one drachm, is a useful purgative; sometimes it is combined with scammony. *Calomel* is too violent in its action to be used safely in most cases; in doses of one to two grains it effectually opens the bowels. *Croton oil*, one to three drops, acts similarly, but is irritant. *Epsom salts* (ʒj to ʒij) is frequently very drastic. Syrup of buckthorn, rhubarb, colocynth, and senna are apt to prove uncertain in their action and cannot be relied upon except as adjuncts. Universal experience seems to have determined that *castor-oil* is the best cathartic for the dog in doses of about half an ounce; and the most convenient routine cathartic is that known as the "Castor-oil mixture," composed as follows :—Ol. Ricini, 3 pts.; Syr. Rham. Cath., 2 pts.; Syr. Papav. Rhe., 1 part." Dose, a dessert to a

---

* Most dogs will lap up castor-oil given in milk.

tablespoonful.* Laxative food, such as vegetable substances, should, when time admits, be given previously to the physic, to gently move on any bones or other hard matters liable to become impacted under the influence of the cathartic.

EMETICS.—We elsewhere deal with the abuse of these important agents. It is to be distinctly understood that they should only be resorted to when we wish to exert a sedative action or to free the stomach from something which is causing or aggravating disease. Thus they are admissible in cases of sedative poisoning, certain forms of epilepsy, and of overgorging with food; and their administration requires the greatest judgment. Our main difficulty is generally to prevent the animal expelling by vomition useful medicines. A *common emetic* is a teaspoonful of salt with half that amount of mustard given in warm water, but there can be no doubt that even this is occasionally dangerously irritant. *Tartar emetic*, a medicine which scarcely affects herbivora, is violent in its action as a sedative and emetic on the dog. However, it is the best agent with which we are acquainted for the latter purposes in doses of one to three grains. *Calomel*, in doses of one and a half to four grains, is emetic, but the action of this agent on the dog is very powerful and it is liable to produce violent purgation or ptyalism.

EXPECTORANTS.—Squills, ipecacuanha, and rhubarb are the best agents of this class.

VERMIFUGES.—*Areca nut*, in doses of one to two drachms mixed with the dog's food just before it is given to him, is an excellent, the best, tæniafuge, and is also said to drive out round-worms. Administered in this way it will be taken freely. *Oil of turpentine* is very prompt in its action as a vermifuge, but its administration is said to be attended with danger. However, mixed with twice its bulk of common oil it may be given safely in doses of a teaspoonful to a dessert-spoonful. Other vermifuges such as *santonin* (gr. j to iij), calomel (gr. j to iij), kousso, hellebore, and filix mas are used occasionally. A vermifuge should always be followed up by a cathartic dose.

STIMULANTS, SEDATIVES, AND NARCOTICS sometimes are very violent in their action on dogs of high nervous temperament, but they prove proportionately valuable in the hands of the skilled practitioner. Opium can be taken in fairly large amounts, the crude gum resin being given in doses of two to four grains, and laudanum from half a drachm to a drachm. Blaine in warning us against adopting human doses for the dog, tells us that "a dog could take without any derangement a dose of opium which would destroy a man; on the contrary, the quantity of nux vomica or crowfig that would destroy the largest dog would fail to destroy a man." Mercurials require the greatest caution in administration to the dog; tobacco given internally or applied externally is apt to cause death; and carbolic acid if applied over an extensive surface affected with mange, or licked by the animal, rapidly and fatally disorganises the blood.

Chloroform, too, requires the greatest caution in its administration to the dog, and probably laughing gas would prove much better suited. In many cases there is a difficulty in obtaining the anæsthetic effects of the drug and the animal does not rally. From experience we may lay down the rule that no animal which is debilitated by disease or with irregular heart's beat should be put under chloroform. It must be remembered that the arguments in favour of the use of ANÆSTHETICS are not nearly so strong in the case of lower animals as in that of man, that we seldom have the necessary skilled assistants available, that in the dog we have not such command over the pulse indications as in man and the larger herbivora, and that chloroform is known to be frequently fatal to the dog. With all due respect to the views of some authors, we are fully of opinion that all minor operations on the dog may be most safely and humanely performed without chloroform. In *giving chloroform to a dog* we must remember how freely he can and does breathe through the mouth. The best method is to hold a sponge on which chloroform has been poured under a cloth loosely thrown over the head of the animal, which is held lying on its side on a table. Gruby has studied the *anæsthetic effects of ether* on dogs. He gives fifty minutes as the maximum and forty seconds as the minimum time required to bring on intoxication which lasted twelve to thirty minutes. Dogs twenty days old lost their sensibility in three minutes, and died in eighteen to twenty minutes; adult dogs lost sensation in eight minutes, and died if the action of the ether was continued for forty-five minutes; copious bleeding recovered young dogs apparently lifeless ('Veterinary Record,' iii, p. 109).

Having thus touched briefly on the leading points to be remembered in canine medicine, administration, and prescription, we may remark that *ordinary and not dangerous remedies may be given in some proportion to the doses for the horse.* Generally in a prescription, grains must be substituted for drachms, and half-fluid drachms for ounces. This rule will be found a useful guide to the student as indicating the maximum limit of doses. A posological table will be found at the end of this work.

The *subcutaneous injection of medicines* has not yet been largely made use of in canine practice, indeed the facility of administration by other methods renders it necessary only in a few cases, and the high nervous temperament of some sick dogs would render the puncture of skin not · altogether free from danger of inducing convulsions.

We must now proceed to make a few remarks about EXTERNAL APPLICATIONS AND MINOR SURGERY. The skin of the dog is readily affected by external stimulants, which, therefore, may be weaker than would be required for the horse by one-fourth. Their application must be followed by prevention of the animal scratching himself and biting the irritated parts. The latter may be effected by means of a wire or perforated tin muzzle, the perforated one having also the advantage that it prevents the patient licking the blistered parts and so suffering from the effects of the cantharides, turpentine, or mercury compound unintentionally ingested. The BLISTER used may be in the form of a *plaster,* ointment, or liquid application; it is applied as for the horse and the usual after-treatment adopted. This method of dealing with cases is specially required among sporting dogs in injuries, tumours, and, most frequently, joint diseases. Mustard plasters, sheep-skin, soap liniment, and other external stimulants familiar to veterinary surgeons are also resorted to in dog practice. FIRING is specially used for greyhounds, and other sporting dogs. The French and Arabs are very fond of it in canine practice. Peuch and Toussaint urge the necessity of firing lightly and with great delicacy by means of a light leaf-shaped cautery with slightly blunted point, heated to a red-brown (about 20° of Daniell's pyrometer). The patient may be placed under the influence of anæsthetics and the hair cut off. Some advocate the use of copper firing irons in dog cases. SETONS are very useful in canine practice, and are generally inserted at the nape of the neck (as in convulsions, chorea, &c.) beneath the throat in coughs, and along the sides in chest diseases. The smallest-sized veterinary seton needle may be used, or one specially manufactured for dog practice with an elliptical cutting head, long narrow shank, and longitudinal eye.

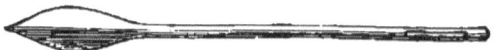

FIG. 9.—Dog seton needle. (PEUCH and TOUSSAINT.)

FOMENTATION presents no special features except that with long-haired dogs great care is necessary to prevent after-chill, and it is not generally advisable to remove the coat. The canine practitioner has a great advantage over the veterinary in that he can resort to the effects of BATHS of various temperatures, which prove most valuable therapeutic means. The *warm bath*, at about 76° Fahr., is specially useful in cases of nervous disorder, internal spasm, fainting, and many other disordered conditions, as an anodyne, antispasmodic, and sedative means. The head must never be submerged. The patient must at once be removed on the occurrence of any signs of weakness, such as panting and a tendency to faint. The bath should not be continued more than ten minutes, and the patient should be rapidly dried to an extent, and then wrapped up in a blanket on removal. Occasionally it will be found that the hot bath proves too much for the animal; he must then be swiftly withdrawn and supported by stimulants.

COLD BATHING AND BANDAGING prove valuable for general or local tonic purposes. The former is specially needed in certain nervous disorders and in atony of the skin, the latter for certain injuries. After bathing or washing of any kind it is well that dogs should have their ears and eyes thoroughly cleansed from soap or water and thoroughly dried, even with greater assiduity than other parts of the body. In dogs with rheumatic or jaundice tendency cold bathing is specially to be avoided, and for routine daily cleansing dry rubbing is to be preferred to washing.

WASHING should not be practised too often, or it will spoil the coat. The yolk of egg is preferable to soap for cleansing the skin of the dog. We owe this useful fact to Mayhew, who smears the yellow well into the hair, pours a little water on to the back and rubs it up into a lather, then clears it off by copious ablutions; but, even if some is left on, the dog will not on its account neglect his personal appearance. The egg does not irritate his eyes and skin as soap does.

BLEEDING of dogs is seldom resorted to in the present day but will occasionally be found useful. It may be performed at the jugular or, less often, at the cephalic and saphena. The dog is first muzzled and then held steady; the vein is opened by means of a small fleam as used for sheep, or of a lancet, after having in the case of the jugular been raised by a ligature around the neck and the hair over the seat of operation having been cut off; 6—12 fluid ounces may be withdrawn, but this is rather too much in most cases, Blaine says one to eight ounces may be taken according to the size of the dog. Chabert agrees that one or two hectogrammes of blood may be withdrawn from a medium-sized dog. The bleeding may be checked by removal of the ligature. Slitting the ear or cutting of the tail are rough means of local bleeding, sometimes resorted to in emergency.

BANDAGING is especially useful in cases of fracture, hernia, and "canker of the ear." Dogs are very liable to shift ordinary bandages, so pitch plaster, plaster of Paris, gutta percha, and starch are used to stiffen and "set" them in cases of fracture or dislocation. Peuch and Toussaint insert a useful illustration of the means of applying some forms of bandage to the dog.

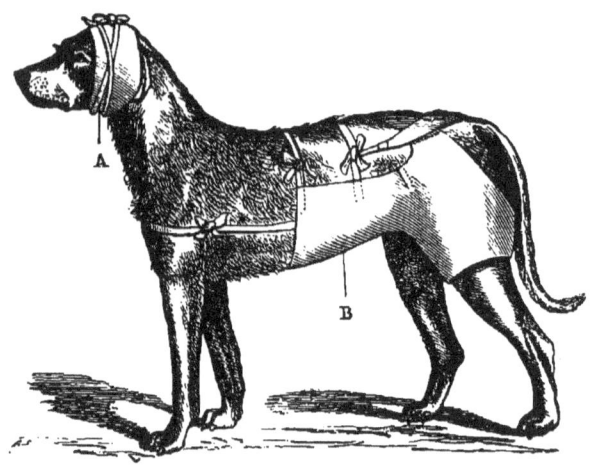

FIG. 10.—A. Bandage des Oreilles v. Béguin. B. Abdominal bandage. (PEUCH and TOUSSAINT.)

MUZZLING is valuable from a surgical point of view as a means of protection of the surgeon and assistants during operations; also to prevent the patient gnawing irritable parts in cases of disease or stimulant applications. The open wire muzzle is the best for general use; occasionally the perforated leather or punctured tin muzzle will be required to prevent licking. The ordinary leather muzzle answers very well in most cases, or a muzzle may be improvised out of an ordinary piece of seton tape by winding it around the nose and securing it as in the accompanying figure, which explains itself.

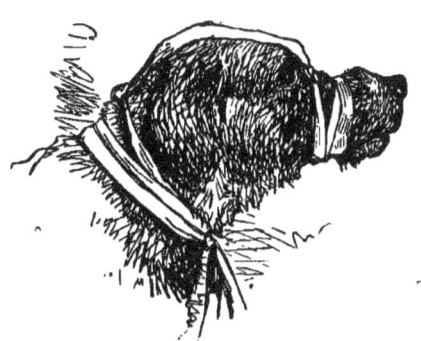

FIG. 11.—Method of fastening tape on a dog's nose to muzzle him.
(MAYHEW.)

The fore legs may need to be tied down by means of a towel to prevent the patient scratching. Big dogs may prove unamenable to reason and so need to be put under the influence of anæsthetics even for minor operations. It is probable that canine operative surgery will in time undergo developments to an extent much exceeding that of veterinary surgery. In dealing with dogs we often have exceptional facilities for nursing and also the patients are freely manipulable, hence the strict application of the *system of antiseptic surgery* is more possible here than in ordinary veterinary surgery. Also the fact that a dog, unlike most larger animals, is generally valued as a friend and companion rather than from a strict pecuniary point of view, gives room for operative interference for simple saving of life without restoration to usefulness, a surgical triumph not likely to lead to thanks from the owner of either a horse or ox in most instances. On the other hand, the domesticated herbivora as a rule require less delicate surgery than does the dog, the parts operated on are much larger, and these patients are much less liable to exaggerated nervous disturbance such as has sometimes to be combated by the canine surgeon.

CHAPTER III.—DISEASES OF THE BLOOD.

THE blood of the dog is estimated to amount to one eighteenth the total weight of the body, its red corpuscles are smaller than those of man. The majority of dogs may be considered as of the sanguine temperament, although the nervous temperament predominates in toy terriers and some of the larger breeds are decidedly lymphatic. These differences materially influence the doses in which medicaments are to be given, and also, to an extent, the remedies to be resorted to in special cases.

The blood diseases of the dog have always been deemed of much importance, even when but two of them were recognised as such, distemper and rabies; but latterly the addition of many others, such as anthrax, diphtheria, foot-and-mouth disease, glanders, and relapsing fever, to the list have rendered this branch of canine pathology specially important. The non-specific blood affections have been comparatively little studied, but they are fairly numerous and very important clinically.

SPECIFIC BLOOD DISORDERS : RABIES.—This formidable disease has a terrible importance from a comparative pathological point of view, since it annually claims human victims in considerable numbers and induces symptoms which, by their severity and the amount of mental disorder which they comprise, excite the greatest apprehension among the friends and onlookers of the case, together with the greatest pity for the sufferer. Rabies has attained a sensational notoriety disproportioned to the actual number of human beings which succumb to it, and which notoriety at times becomes almost morbidly exaggerated, indeed so much so as to impress excessively nervous and hysterical persons with the severest apprehension, inducing symptoms almost resembling those of the disease. An average amount of notoriety is a decided advantage as ensuring the necessary legislative and other measures required for the repression of rabies, which otherwise would make headway, to the detriment of man and all kinds of domesticated animals, no species of which, quadruped or bird, is capable of resisting inoculation with rabid virus. As we wish to deal with this disease especially on a sound *practical* basis, we shall in turn deal with its diagnosis and its prevention. We may preface these divisions of our subject by saying a little about the other matters which require notice in a systematic record of a disease.

The *symptoms* of rabies should be examined only in so far as is required for diagnosis, and can be ascertained with safety to the observer and the public. Responsibility lies with anyone who having a dog which he knows to be "mad" keeps him alive and so runs the risk of his escaping and injuring the public.* This disease has hitherto resisted curative treatment so obstinately that in ordinary cases destruction of the patient should *at once* follow exact diagnosis. This is a sound principle to go on, with the distinct reservation that probably, in the future, science will throw light on the treatment of specific disorders to bring about *cure*, whereas she now can but insist on *prevention*. We must leave the *geography* and *history* of the disorder to be perused in such works as Fleming's on 'Rabies and Hydrophobia,' where the subject is thoroughly dealt with. Thus there remains for our consideration the question of how to determine the disease when present and how to prevent its occurrence and extension.

DIAGNOSIS.—Dogs affected with rabies differ much in their mode of manifesting the disorder, such differences depending to an extent on the habits of the animal in health. These varieties in the symptoms have led canine

* As has been legally established by a ruling of Lord Kenyon quoted by Youatt, 'The Dog,' p. 153.

pathologists to consider that every strangeness in behaviour of a dog is to be observed with suspicion; and Bouley has established the rule of always looking at a sick dog with apprehension, especially one which seems too fond of you, considering him to be rabid until proved otherwise. It so often happens that dangerously rabid animals but not known to be mad are brought by their owners for medicinal treatment that this rule cannot be too strictly enforced. It is remarkable that in rabies the owner is the last person to whom the animal is inclined to be aggressive, and, moreover, in certain cases the patient is excessively affectionate, licking the hands and face of his mistress, which practice has in many recorded instances conveyed the disease, especially when a pimple or other small wound has been on the licked part. The popular idea that a mad dog is furious is correct only as concerns certain forms of the disease. In the furious form paroxysms of rage are well marked, and are especially excited by the sight of strange dogs or the glistening of light on the surface of water. The violence of these paroxysms exhausts the animal, so that between them he dozes or sleeps soundly, but if disturbed awakens in a fury. The wrath of the patient varies in different individuals and stages of disease; it either assumes the form of a blind fury, prompting the dog to fly at and worry any strange object, such as a stick inserted through the bars of his cage, or there seems a sort of "method in his madness," which has been considered an "instinctive desire to propagate the affection"; thus dogs are the special object of aversion, and cats, too, excite the animal to fury, but later herbivora and then men come on the list of those to whom he will do mischief. It is remarked that in the case of rabid herbivora the greatest fury is felt towards dogs, and this is sometimes seen in the case of human beings. The fury is preceded by a period of strange restlessness, a quickness and irritability of the temper, and sometimes a remarkable amount of treachery. The animal is dull but watchful, and a very characteristic symptom is a tendency to snap at flies or other real or imaginary objects, after watching their course for a little time, as though to obtain a favorable opportunity for the act of aggression. While dozing between the paroxysms the animal often starts up suddenly and wildly.

Manifestations of irksomeness of restraint occur early in the case, and the mad dog will show the greatest cunning in getting loose. Having done so, he will traverse enormous distances and finally return home, if he has escaped the various dangers of his journey, in a thoroughly exhausted, perhaps paralysed, condition. The pace adopted is a slow, dogged sort of trot; at first the

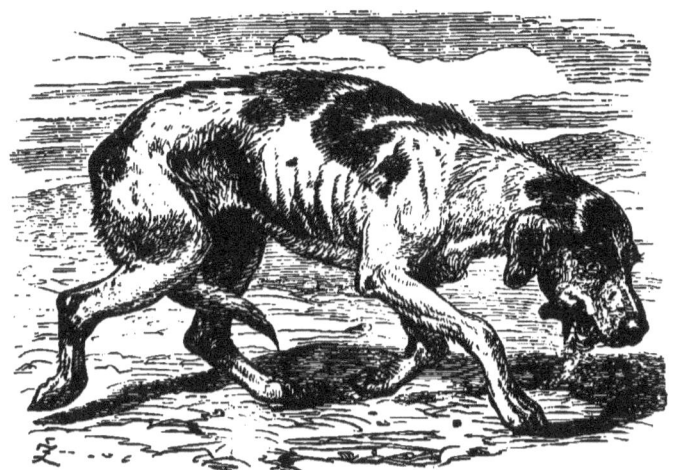

Fig 12.—Figure of mad dog (furious stage). After SANSON.

animal may go from side to side, evidently intending mischief to creatures met by him on his track, but soon he goes straight forward, attacking only when opposed, in a state of semi-stupor, his movements becoming uncertain in consequence of the combined effects of weariness and imminent paralysis. The furious animal is very sudden in his attacks, the unprovoked nature and *élan* of which overawe the assaulted animal, which is simply rolled over if small enough, and bitten by one or two snaps, and left in the search for a fresh victim. In this way an incredibly large number of sheep may be injured by one dog in a very short time. It has been supposed that sound dogs manifest an instinctive aversion to rabid ones, but such is not the case, as has been amply proved. The unfortunate tendency of mad dogs to travel great distances, especially during the night, has much increased the belief in the spontaneous origin of this disease; the animal which brought it into the neighbourhood having passed through and done the mischief unobserved. Numerous cases of this kind are on record where very strict inquiries have proved instances of supposed spontaneity to be, really, unobserved inoculation. The mad dog is characterised by his contempt for threats and his fearlessness; this is partly due to perverted or lost sensation and partly to mental perversion, which latter seems in some cases in the dog, as in hydrophobic men, associated with a remarkable degree of self-restraint, so that the hand will be seized with apparent fury, but freed without infliction of a wound after being retained in the mouth and champed for a little while. The question of whether or no this mental aversion extends to the fear of water in the dog and the supervention of paroxysms at the sound of falling water, as in man, has been much discussed, because it was thought that the fear of water would be a sound and easily applied test for diagnosis of rabies in the dog. Suffice it to say that it has been amply established that this is not a pathognomonic symptom, and is altogether insufficient as a test. The rabid animal will approach water freely and drink when not prevented by spasm of the throat or the loss of swallowing power seen in the latter stages; even then, however, he will endeavour to slake his almost insatiable thirst. The mouth becomes very dry and of a dark purple colour after the disease has been present for some time, and in the "dumb" form the lower jaw drops and the throat is swollen (a symptom which disappears at death). Occasionally the whole head is œdematous, generally the tongue is pendulous, it often has been injured, and the teeth, especially the canines, may have been broken by the furious attempts of the animal to escape from con-

DISEASES OF THE BLOOD. 31

finement or to destroy hard objects. In the early stages there is profuse salivation, but this does not last longer than a couple of days; a small amount of froth may collect at the angles of the mouth, and the patient endeavours to remove it by rubbing with the paws. The animal in such cases is generally supposed to have a bone in the throat, a report which must be always looked upon with the greatest suspicion as probably dumb rabies. Only in the earliest stages is vomition present, and a small amount of blood may be expelled; later there is paralysis of the alimentary canal, as indicated by obstinate constipation and the tendency of foreign bodies to accumulate in the pharynx and stomach. Such foreign matters as straws, sticks, and hair are picked up by the dog in the earliest stages of the disorder, when there is perverted appetite as indicated by appreciation of anything cold to the tongue when licked, by tendency to eat dung, either his own or that of other dogs, horses, &c., also to lap urine (which is considered very diagnostic). As paralysis of the throat sets in, the ingested matters are retained at the back of the mouth against or in the pharynx. Male dogs are most often affected, probably because there are more of them, and not on account of any special sexual features, or deprivation of opportunity for sexual gratification simultaneously with high excitement, as was at one time supposed. It has been observed, but not proved, that when a pregnant female has been bitten, any active manifestation of the effects of inoculation is reserved until after parturition has taken place, then the bitch may for a time perform well her duties as a mother, but it is possible, although not proved, that she may convey the disease to her offspring in her milk. Fever is present in rabies, and in the more advanced stages there is a hollow sound in breathing, which act is especially performed through the nose. The eye of the mad dog is at times abnormally bright and red, and may present a certain amount of strabismus, which gives the animal an excessively sinister appearance; in other cases (especially of the dumb form of the disease) the eyes are dull, sad, and heavy looking, and, very occasionally, there is an accumulation of pus at the inner angle, and simultaneously there is a purulent discharge from the nostrils. The dull appearance of the eyes, generally distressed appearance, pendulous tongue and lower jaw, dark colour of the tongue, and dry state of the mouth, give the animal a very diagnostic appearance in the dumb form, in which the disease runs its course with special rapidity, and there is a marked tendency to the early supervention of paralysis preceded by twitchings and stiffness. In this way the face, back, and hind limbs are successively invaded, and at last the animal becomes thoroughly paralysed.

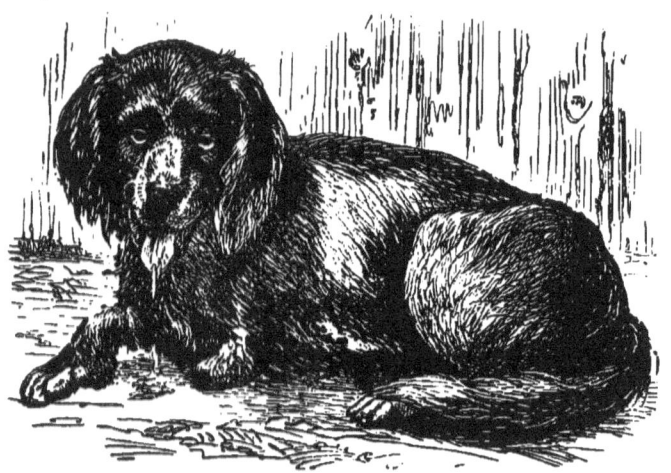

Fig. 13.—Figure of mad dog (dumb form). After Sanson.

Apart from the gastric derangement above alluded to, the digestive organs are sometimes the seat of spasm, and the animal may collect the straw of his bed underneath his belly and press on it, apparently in the hope to relieve the abdominal pain. It has been noticed that when the digestive canal is affected the case proves rapidly fatal. In the early phases of the disorder sexual excitement is common, and bitches are much less liable to be bitten than dogs; it has been observed in dog-packs of hounds that one of the earliest symptoms is a tendency to lick the anus and generative organs of another dog. Another warning symptom noticed especially early among hounds has been an alteration in the voice; the howl of a mad dog must be heard to be realised and once heard will never be forgotten; any description will necessarily be insufficient to convey its true characters, but it has been spoken of as an imperfect bark followed by a series of incompleted howls, the animal being seated on his rump with the muzzle elevated in the air and often turned backwards while it rests against the wall. Another symptom of great diagnostic value is the tendency of the animal to constantly lick or, later, bite and lacerate with the teeth some one part of the body, the seat of the inoculation wound which may be found in a green gangrenous state or merely a scar. The persistence of irritation at the seat of injury, or its recurrence with pathological changes after the wounds have apparently healed, is one of the most remarkable of the many extraordinary facts about rabies. It has led to the belief that the virus is not absorbed, but remains at the seat of injury, and there undergoes changes which render it capable of affecting the system in general; on this is based the practice of excision of the parts around the wound as a preventive at any time before active manifestation of symptoms. Blaine was firmly convinced of the benefit of such excision, but it cannot be accepted as conclusively proved that rabies may thus be prevented. However, active measures adopted with every evidence of thorough confidence in their efficacy are specially necessary in dealing with dogbite in mankind, for people if not thoroughly convinced that they are out of danger are apt to work themselves into a serious semi-hysterical state closely resembling actual hydrophobia. In the dog rabies proves invariably fatal, the cases lasting from three to seven days when allowed to pursue their natural course. Even after death diagnosis is often a matter of importance; the canine surgeon may be called on to give an opinion about the emaciated bedraggled carcass of an unfortunate animal which has been killed after being run down in the public streets, or of some less bruised and injured dog which has been more humanely but injudiciously destroyed after infliction of a bite on its owner or someone who has had to do with it. Such revengeful slaughter or prompt destruction with a view to prevent accidents is an error of judgment, for if the dog had been kept alive with due precautions his freedom from rabies might be established on the clearest evidence, and thus the apprehensions of persons bitten thoroughly allayed; for it is almost certain that *no animal free from rabies, however angry he be, can give another animal or man rabies by a bite.* The dog should be kept alive in order that it may be thoroughly established that rabies was not incubating in his system. The incubation of the disorder in the dog varies from a week to a year, but it is highly probable that only during the time immediately preceding and during active manifestations of the symptoms is it that the saliva is virulent. Therefore keeping the animal alive for a short time, say a fortnight, should suffice to prove whether he was in a condition to convey the disease. It must be remembered that the body of a dog in the latter stages of incubation would present no definite and absolutely distinctive lesions of rabies. However, when the disease has set in there are some *abnormalities detectable post mortem* which amply suffice for diagnosis. Even in a body considerably advanced in decomposition (such as has sometimes to be examined in this relation) the accumulation of foreign bodies, generally of a nature not to readily decompose, will be detectable in the stomach and at the back of the mouth. In fresher cases the respiratory and alimentary tracts should be examined with the greatest care, as also the central organs of the nervous system (cerebro-spinal), both macroscopically and microscopically. Increased vascularity, a streaky congestion, is found at the base of the tongue and sometimes invading the whole of the fauces, especially the tonsils. The upper part of the larynx also, is a frequent seat of this lesion, and the whole lining membrane of the trachea may be congested, or, in severe cases, spotted. In the larynx the membrane about the epiglottis is specially liable to be affected, and the pharynx is more or less involved. It has been remarked that the raging form of the disease is specially characterised by respiratory lesions, even the costal pleura and diaphragm being affected in some cases, whereas in the dumb form the changes are most marked throughout the alimentary canal. The salivary glands are congested, and the lining membrane of the stomach, and to a variable extent also of the intestines, is the seat of spots of extravasated blood and streaky stagnation; also we may find sphacelated ulcerated patches or extravasations of blood between the coats of the stomach, and Blaine speaks of the mucous membrane as "not unfrequently sprinkled over with pustular prominences." Adhesions of the peritoneum and intussusception are often present. The body rapidly decays. The contents of the stomach are, in addition to the usual accumulation of indigestible substances, merely a small amount of coffee-coloured material, apparently extravasated blood altered in colour and characters by the digestive juices. In this, as in almost all other blood diseases, petechiæ may be found in any or every of the tissues, as the peritoneum, mediastinum, or substance of the heart. The meninges of the brain (especially the pia mater), and of the spinal cord at its anterior extremity, show an exceptional amount of congestion which the substance of the enclosed nerve masses also occasionally shares. The arachnoid and subarachnoid fluids are generally somewhat increased in quantity. The lymphatic glands throughout the body, and the spleen and liver are generally found enlarged and congested. Such are the most frequent and constant lesions detectable on nakedeye examination of the carcases of rabid animals. The degree of blood extravasation varies in different cases, being sometimes excessive and sometimes with difficulty detectable, the lining membrane of stomach, endocardium, and brain are the most frequent seat of extensive escape of blood. The conditions of the stomach, its contents, of the larynx, fauces, and base of the tongue are most useful for diagnostic purposes. Inflammations of various parts are described as present in this disease, but the correctness of this pathological statement has not been established. In the critical post-mortem examination it must not be forgotten to record absence of any morbid condition which might give rise to symptoms such as could be mistaken for those of rabies, nor to note the state of the tongue and teeth, whether injured or intact, nor the state of the eyes, body in general, and any evidences of severe injury. It is probable that some of the latter have been entered in published accounts of the morbid anatomy of rabies. Siedamgrotzsky ('Bericht über d. Veterinärwesen in Sachsen,'* 1874) has recorded his special observations of the rare cases in which the eyes undergo morbid changes† in true rabies such as make the case liable to be confounded with distemper. These changes are essentially degenerative, such as moderate cell-heaping in the vicinity of the ulcers which form, fatty degeneration of the corneal elements, and opening out of the interstitial substance. The ulcer progresses rapidly, and may lead to complete perforation, and escape of the aqueous humour, or this may be prevented by a thin layer of fibrin or a blood-clot in the anterior chamber. Siedamgrotzsky found these changes in only six cases; he does not attribute them to injury, but to trophic alterations due to the nervous lesions of the affection.

The changes in the central nervous organs detectable by means of the microscope have been variously described by different observers. Coats ('Royal Med. and Chir. Society,' Dec. 11th, 1877) found an aggregation of leucocytes around the medium sized vessels of the spinal cord, medulla oblongata, pons Varolii, and corpora quadrigemina, the smallest being in the convolutions. These aggregations are similar to those detectable in the salivary glands and mucous follicles of the larynx. He concludes that the lesions are very like those of tetanus, and that both

* Vide 'Veterinary Journal,' October, 1876.
† Youatt, especially, noted deep-seated ulceration in the eye in some cases of rabies.

disorders are due to blood poisons affecting the central nervous system and remarkably nearly identical localities, the irritation seeming to centre in the medulla oblongata, as probably determined by the anatomical and physiological relations of the nutrient vessels. Dr. Gowers had found in the medulla in hydrophobia not only leucocytes around the blood-vessels but also an infiltration of the tissues with them, forming in places groups which might be termed miliary abscesses. Kolessnikow, of the Veterinary Institute of St. Petersburgh, found the small veins distended with white corpuscles, their walls infiltrated with similar elements, and the endothelial cells of the intima of the veins and capillaries proliferating freely, as also did the connective tissue cells of the adventitia. He also found a clear, yellowish, refractive substance between the endothelial cells and adventitia and inner coat, rarely in the lumen. These changes were especially well marked in the parietal and frontal lobes of the cerebral hemispheres, but were also found in other parts. Infiltration of the walls of the vessels was especially seen in the medulla oblongata. Changes were noted around the deep-seated origins of the hypoglossal, spinal accessory, and vagus nerves. The spinal canal was usually plugged with a granular mass and surrounded by lymphoid elements. Recent researches show the "leucocytes" or lymphoid cells of these observers to be bacteria.

Among the other brilliant discoveries made by M. Pasteur recently, has been his observation that rabies may be communicated by inoculation with substance of the cerebral cortex, of the medulla oblongata, and with the cerebro-spinal fluid. By trephining a healthy dog and placing in contact with its brain cerebral tissue from an animal affected with either form of rabies, the disease may be conveyed *with certainty in a few days.* This method has been applied to rabbits and other harmless animals as a diagnostic means; Gibier uses fowls, and considers that they recover from the disease spontaneously; he describes a special bacterium of rabies, but his views have not been accepted by Pasteur.

In *the differential diagnosis of rabies* a number of popular errors as regards the disease have to be avoided. Thus extensive frothing from the mouth, fear of water, constant firm compression of the tail between the hind legs are not seen in this disease so invariably as to make them pathognomonic. Also the presence of ranula, or cysts beneath the tongue, which used to be insisted on, is not to be relied on. It has been supposed that bitches never turn mad spontaneously, but then we do not know that dogs do so either; certain it is that spaying as a preventive of rabies is a fallacy, although it seems to be rather extensively resorted to in France. That dogs which have been "wormed" do not go mad, and that removal of the tip of an animal's tail, taking care that one of the tendons of the depressors is drawn out and shall curl up like a worm in elastic recoil when broken, are ideas based on ignorance but not yet obsolete. The occasional occurrence of a pustular discharge from the nose and eyes with corneal ulceration in rabies have sometimes led to confusion of this disease with distemper, yet the differences between the two disorders are so marked as to render such a mistake possible only with very careless diagnosis. Fits due to epilepsy, especially those which follow distemper, differ altogether from symptoms shown in rabies. The rabid dog does not lose consciousness, he does not lie on the ground struggling and champing the jaws and foaming at the mouth as an epileptic does; the latter may on "coming to" bite anyone holding him and rush off, but his escape is very different from the way in which the mad dog "runs a muck." Youatt speaks of cases where dogs have been bitten on the ear and the disease thus conveyed been mistaken for canker of the ear; in each the irritable part will be energetically scratched, but in rabies some of the earlier symptoms of general disorder will be present at this stage, and there will be no such local eruptions as are found in ear canker; tetanus, colic, and (as we have already seen) bone in the throat have been confused in diagnosis with rabies. Such errors can occur only with imperfect examination of the case. The practitioner must never arrive at conclusions hastily, he must, with due precautions, thoroughly examine the animal and not decide that rabies is present without ample evidence in support of this view.

For the seizure of mad dogs several mechanical means have been devised, one of which is shown in Peuch and Toussaint's 'Surgery;' the figures of these will explain themselves.

FIG. 14.—Pince collier pour saisir le Chien. (After PEUCH and TOUSSAINT.)

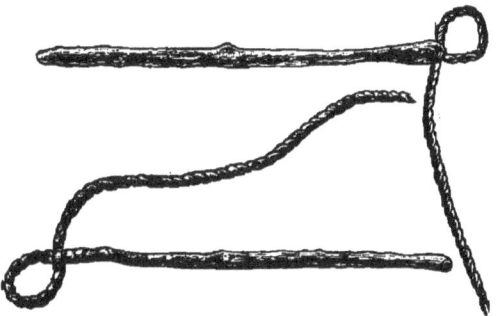

FIG. 15.—Bouley's sticks and rope.

It must be remembered that the disease has been conveyed by saliva smeared over the coat,* by the face of a human being having been licked by a mad dog, and even by still more obscure methods. Thus Dr. Evans, in the 'Journal of the United Service Institution of India' for 1883 (July), mentions a case of fatal hydrophobia in a tanner, traceable to currying the skin of a cow which died from rabies in London, Canada West, in 1866. In making *post-mortem examinations of the carcases of mad dogs* every precaution should be observed, although it has been

* Galtier has shown that rabific saliva remains virulent in drinking-water even twenty-four hours after the diseased dog has tried to drink. This source of possible conveyance of the disease should be carefully avoided.

accepted that virulence does not persist in the carcass twenty-four hours after death. The autopsy should not be performed by anyone with sores on the hands; the bodies of rabid animals should be disposed of by thorough and complete destruction by means of fire or quicklime. Similar precautions should be taken with the carcases of rabid animals of species other than the canine, the several fluids and tissues of which have been found just as virulent as those of the dog, although the liability of the patient to communicate the disease varies in direct relation to his natural normal ferocity. These measures of precaution may seem too elaborate for prevention of a disease the spontaneity of which has not been proved, and which in 98 per cent. of the cases which occur is directly traceable to a bite; but it should be remembered that our knowledge of disease-producing agents and their modes of diffusion, although much increased of late years, is as yet open to great expansion, and every carcass of an animal which has succumbed to specific disorder should be looked on with apprehension as a possible centre of communication and diffusion of the disease.

Rabies seems to differ somewhat in accordance with geographical range, just as anthrax and other important specific disorders are known to do. Dr. Colam, writing to the 'Veterinary Journal,' describes the dog disease of the Arctic regions. It broke out about 1859 and spread over nearly the whole of North Greenland. It is communicable from dog to fox but there is no record of its communication to man, yet the natives have a horror of being bitten by an affected animal, although they use the skin and even eat the flesh occasionally. The Danish Government has circulated official directions for prophylaxis. On post-mortem examination a pitchy substance is found in the intestines and ulceration for four inches on either side of the ilio-cæcal valve. This disease is the same probably as occurred in Dr. Hayes' expedition to Smith's Sound in 1866-67, and Nares' expedition in 1875-76. Dr. Kane in 1854 observed in the Arctic regions a disease the symptoms of "which so closely resembled rabies as to cause alarm," such as avoidance of water, drinking with aversion and spasm, and staggering gait, head depressed, and mouth foaming and tumid, also snappishness. The sunless Arctic winter is supposed to be the cause of an anomalous form of disease, "as clearly mental as in the case of any human being. The material functions of the poor brutes go on without interruption; they eat voraciously, retain their strength, and sleep well. But all the indications beyond this go to prove that the original epilepsy, which was the first manifestation of brain disease among them, has been followed by a true lunacy. They barked frenzically at nothing and walked in straight and curved lines with anxious and unwearying perseverance. They fawn on you, but without seeming to appreciate the notice you give them in return, pushing their heads against your person, or oscillating with a strange pantomime of fear. Their most intelligent actions seem automatic. Sometimes they remain for hours in moody silence, and then start off howling as if pursued, and run up and down for hours." A strong tendency to tonic spasm, attributed to lengthened cold and darkness, affected both men and dogs. In the latter it assumed the form of tetanus, and carried off fifty-seven of them with symptoms not unlike those of hydrophobia ('Arctic Explorations,' quoted by Fleming). Rabies has been observed to assume some special features in some parts of North America; thus we read of the "Californian Dog Disease." Walley has pointed out some of its peculiarities in Edinburgh. It most frequently assumed the dumb form and was seen in well-bred dogs, strange to say, fresh cases were most frequent on Saturday, Sunday, and Monday. Hiccough, a very rare phenomenon in dogs, occurred in one or two cases. The temperature was noted as 104·5° Fahr. in the earlier stages, very low in the late stages, in one or two instances below 95°. It was most liable to be confounded with cerebro-spinal meningitis, a sequela of distemper. Intravenous injection served to prolong life ('Veterinary Journal').

From time to time specific remedies for rabies have

been extensively vaunted, and to an extent accepted by the medical profession, but all have sooner or later been found inefficacious; thus, Blaine and Youatt were inclined to agree with the ancients as to the value of the box tree; Youatt speaks favorably of scutellaria; curara has been thought of value, and cases have recovered under its use. These specifics have temporarily enjoyed reputations not only as curatives, but as prophylactics, and have been found about as valuable for the latter purpose as spaying, worming, or extraction of the tendon of the tail. Eliminative treatment has proved equally ineffectual with specifics. The actual and immediate cause of the disorder is a blood poison (probably Gibier's micrococcus), without which no case of rabies can occur. Our efforts must, therefore, be directed to limiting its range. We know some facts about this poison which tend to the encouragement of future research with a view to rendering the constitutions of animals unfitted for its development and propagation. Thus, although none of the elaborate experiments which have been made to generate rabies spontaneously by exposure to heat, cold, ungratified sexual desire, and so on, have succeeded, and although the old idea of there being certain seasons (known as " dog days ") when as the result of heat the disease prevails especially, it is certain that some years and in certain places the disease assumes an enzootic or epizootic form. Moreover, all animals bitten by mad dogs and untreated do not go mad, even many dogs entirely resist the disease. Also in different cases the period of incubation varies very considerably, and the disease assumes two distinct forms in the dog, the furious being especially the variety in young dogs, whereas the dumb form is seldom seen except in adults. Thus the action of the poison is influenced by constitution, and Pasteur considers that he has devised a method of *rabies inoculation* by which the disease may be prevented or cured. This method has been tested by a French Commission of Scientists which has accepted M. Pasteur's conclusions, which are, therefore, as well substantiated as they can possibly be until time and the practical experience of several generations shall have submitted them to as thorough a test as the Jennerian system of vaccination has been able to stand successfully. Pasteur, Chamberland, and Roux find that the virus transferred from the dog to the ape, and cultivated by propagation through several members of the latter order, becomes progressively feebler after each inoculation. After a certain period of such cultivation, if it be hypodermically administered to dogs, guinea-pigs, or rabbits, even by intracranial injection (the most deadly method), death does not result, but the animal acquires an immunity from hydrophobia. If, on the other hand, the poison of rabies be cultivated in successive rabbits, or guinea-pigs only, its potency is intensified, and after a time is so great that a fatal issue invariably follows its inoculation. The poison as found in the dog is intermediate in strength between that of the two methods of cultivation just mentioned. Thus, by careful selection of the medium, and the stage of cultivation, it is possible to accumulate a store of attenuated virus, which can be relied on to communicate a modified rabies, whose inoculation shall be protective against its severer forms as that of vaccinia is against variola. Since these results were obtained Pasteur has shown with regard to the virus of rabies that it affects the spinal cord before the medulla oblongata; it has its seat in *all* parts of the nervous system; may be retained with all its virulence in the brain and cord for several weeks by freezing or by exclusion of air. This virus has not yet been found associated with any special microbe, it does not seem to be attenuated by cold, and in different species of animals comes to vary greatly in strength and properties when, by successive inoculations, the virus has attained the fixity proper to each genus. Pasteur has different kinds of rabies virus of which he is able to exactly prognosticate the action on special species. He believes that one of these serves to secure immunity to dogs virulently inoculated. He has twenty-three dogs thus rendered insusceptible of rabies. The hypothesis of the passage of the virus from the bite through the nervous system from the periphery is not entirely correct; some virus enters the circulation—although intravenous or intracellular inoculation ordinarily produces "dumb madness," furious rabies will follow when the amount of virus injected is very small, and the smaller the amount the more easily is the furious rabies brought on. In a subsequent communication we find it stated that "by a few transmissions of the virus from monkey to monkey there can be easily obtained a virus so attenuated as shall never communicate, by hypodermic inoculations, the disease to a dog. Inoculations by trepanning of such virus will likewise produce no result; but an animal will, notwithstanding, be rendered thereby proof against the disease. The virulence of the virus becomes, on the contrary, augmented in its passage from rabbit to rabbit."

Such is the basis of the important Pasteurean system for rabies vaccination of dogs, as applied to mankind his methods have attained much notoriety. It is evident that we must for the present rely on the other methods of repressing the disease which have been suggested by experience. Extermination of the whole race of dogs would not suffice for the eradication of rabies, even if such an extensive measure were practicable, for it has been amply proved that cats, also jackals, foxes, skunks,* wolves, and other wild animals, convey the disease. Something may, however, be done, especially in large towns, by causing the number of homeless dogs, such as are little under supervision and so may pass unnoticed

---

* Col. Dodge in his 'Hunting Grounds of the Great West,' says that skunk bites (generally on a sleeping man) are invariably followed by hydrophobia, although the skunk is not necessarily himself affected. This singularly fatal result of skunk-bite is supposed to be confined to the Arkansas Valley ('Veterinary Journal,' vol. v). These opinions must be taken with much reserve. Hovey considers hydrophobia from skunk-bites a different form from that caused by dog-bite, and terms it rabies mephitica. He considers the generation of the poison possibly associated with inactivity of the anal glands and with development of poisonous matter in the mouth follicles. He suggests that the mephitic secretion may be a natural antidote to the salivary virus ('Forest and Stream').

through dangerous stages of the disease, working mischief unobserved, to be lessened by painless slaughter after a definite detention in a Dogs' Home whereby the owners of dogs may have a fair chance of reclaiming favourites or useful animals which have strayed or been lost. Dogs' homes require to be most carefully supervised and worked on sound principles, lest they become centres for diffusion of disease. Quarantine is rendered unsatisfactory by the indefiniteness of the period of incubation of the disease, although a period of six months' strict quarantine would give most cases full opportunity for development, we have no guarantee that all inoculated animals would thereby be detected. Australia is at present endeavouring to secure quarantine of imported dogs, and so to ensure continued freedom from rabies which would, doubtless, spread with terrible rapidity among the dingoes or wild dogs, but quarantine, to be effectual, will require to be supplemented by other methods. Perhaps, in the future, Pasteur's system will ensure immunity; Gibier has found that birds which have once recovered from rabies resist future attacks. Although neither " stamping out " nor quarantine can be relied on as a means of extermination of this disease, they are both valuable means of repression. There can be no doubt that the measures adopted in many large cities for the incarceration or destruction of ownerless dogs, dog taxes, enforced wearing of collars with the owner's name on, diffusion of popular information as to the detection of rabies, and the combating of popular errors on the subject, are of great value in limiting the range of this formidable disorder, and they should be encouraged as much as possible and the Legislature advised to insist on them. Statistics of prevalence of rabies should be carefully prepared, and the disease considered one of the most important to be dealt with by the authorities. That it has not been included in the Contagious Diseases (Animals) Act is a very extraordinary and serious omission, which ought at once to be rectified. No breed of dog should be specially subjected to supervision on account of rabies; authorities are by no means agreed as to the kind in which the disease is most often seen. Youatt has found it most frequently in curs and lurchers, and speaks of it being most often communicated to horses by Dalmatians. Mayhew, whose practice lay among toy and other fancy breeds, considered them most liable; whole packs of foxhounds have had to be destroyed on account of it; Esquimaux sledge-dogs succumb to the disorder, and the Indian pariah dog diffuses it through the country, causing deaths of such valuable animals as horses, elephants, camels, and oxen, in addition to an annual fatality among mankind. It is evident that *muzzling* cannot be universal, and there-

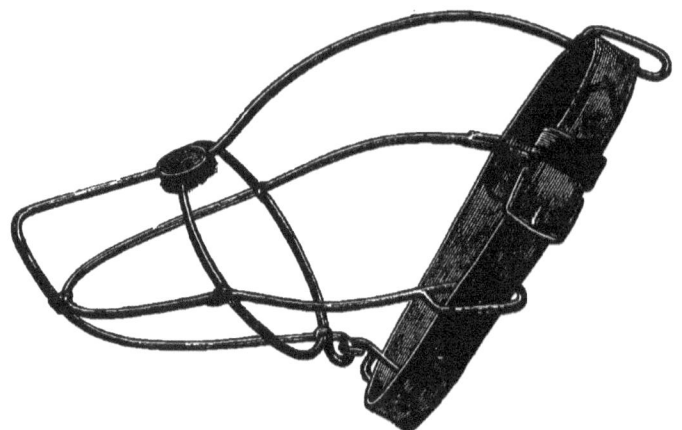

FIG. 16.—Wire muzzle. (After FLEMING).

fore, although beneficial to an extent, cannot be absolutely relied on to prevent outbreaks of the disorder; for dogs which have been bitten by others which are naturally ferocious, or which have been behaving at all strangely or been sick, the muzzle should be used, that made of wire being the least inconvenient to the animal and most humane. *Blunting dogs' teeth*, as specially recommended by M. Bourrel, is no more reliable as thoroughly effectual than muzzling, but still has a limited value which would sanction its adoption under certain circumstances. A muzzle must be removed for the animal to feed, but blunt teeth

DISEASES OF THE BLOOD. 47

are permanently lessened in their power of causing wounds. To perform the operation the mouth is kept open by means of a gag, the tips of the canines are snipped off with small shears, and then the incisors and canines are rounded with a small rasp.

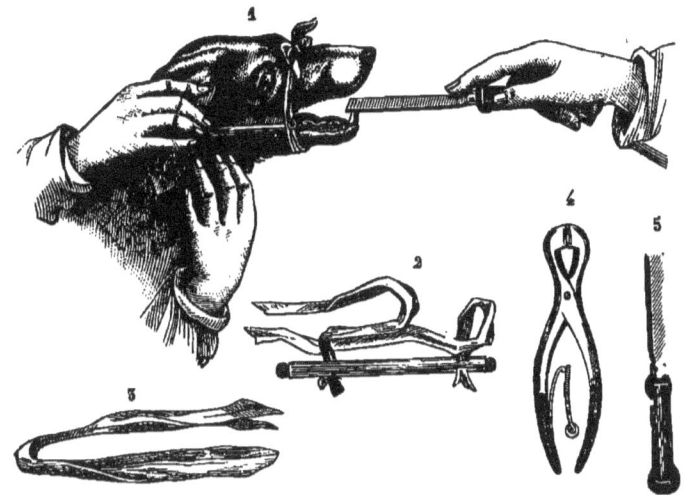

FIG. 17.—Bourrel's rasp and gag for teeth. (PEUCH and TOUSSAINT.)
(1) The operation. (2) The gag. (3) Tape. (4) Shears. (5) Rasp.

In cases where a bite has actually been inflicted, and it has been proved that the inflictor was mad, or he may reasonably be considered dangerous, no time should be lost in dealing vigorously with the wounds. If the victim be a dog (and has not since bitten a man) he should be destroyed, if of little value, rather than run the risks of retaining him alive, because dogs of all animals are the creatures opposing least constitutional resistance to the rabies virus, and they are among the most dangerous because of their predatory instincts as carnivora. When there are urgent arguments against destruction, the bitten animal should, with the greatest care, be thoroughly examined, in order to make sure that all his wounds are detected and treated; he may even need to be shaved for this purpose. The wounds having been treated by excision and cautery, he should be carefully washed and then must be isolated for at least two months (five or six weeks being the average incubation in dogs), and wear the wire muzzle when out of doors, and be kept under supervision (and promptly isolated on any sign of disorder of any kind or strangeness of temper) for at least one year. Few dogs will be worth the risk and solicitude necessitated in these precautions. *The chances against the animal developing the disease after a bite* are—(1) The inflictor of the bite may not be rabid, but if he be, (2) his teeth may have been thoroughly cleaned from morbific saliva by frequent bites of other animals or through clothing; (3) the bitten animal may be constitutionally fitted to resist the disease, (4) or the treatment of the wound as adopted may be effectual in destruction of the virus, (5) or the free flow of blood from the wound as inflicted may suffice to wash away the virus, especially if the flow has been encouraged by suction or cupping. *When a human being has been bitten the following measures may be taken* :—Suction of the wounds by some individual whose mouth is free from abrasions; encouragement of free bleeding from the wounds; neglect of no wound, however apparently trivial, in which the cuticle has become abraded; application of ligature or tourniquet above the seat of injury; prompt application of caustic, especially the nitrate of silver or caustic potash, butter of antimony, or the actual or galvano-cautery. In deep wounds this must be followed by excision all round the injury, taking care never to actually cut into the wound, and to wipe the knife after each stroke, then cauterise the fresh wound thus produced. It is advisable to repeat application of the cautery after separation of the first eschar. These measures, if carefully carried out, should be considered as practically ensuring immunity from ill effects and absolutely sufficient to allay alarm on the part of the patient and his friends. Such measures as bleeding, the cold bath, allowing a stream of water to fall from a height on the wound, and so on, must never be deemed sufficient. The duty of the canine practitioner in dealing with rabies is a

DISEASES OF THE BLOOD. 49

difficult one, for it comprises the constant excitement of apprehension of the Legislature to secure adequate measures of repression, and the simultaneous insistance on the considerable chance of escape of individuals unhappily bitten.

DISTEMPER is, of the numerous diseases to which canine flesh is heir, that which annually exacts the largest tribute of fatality. It is a specific disorder; very wide spread in its prevalence, and supposed to have become domiciled in Great Britain within the last century, but of this we have no absolute proof. It resembles, to an extent, those specific disorders of other animals which are known as "influenza," but it seems to be a distinct and special

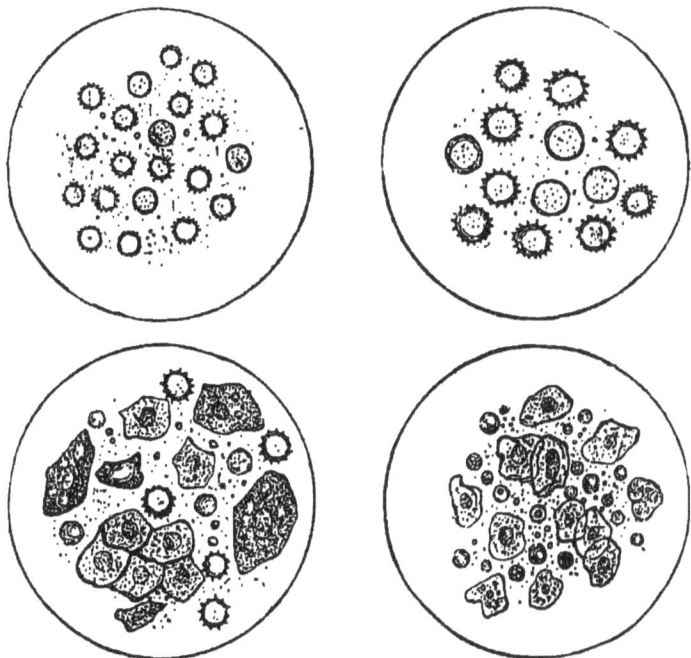

FIGS. 18—21.—Distemper organisms intermingled with various cells.
(After Kreijewski.)

disease, and not the pathological equivalent of any known disorder of man or other animals. An attempt has been made to demonstrate that it is similar to human typhoid,

4

but unsuccessfully, and the same result has followed comparison of it with influenza of the horse and strangles. Possibly through confusion between this disease and true variola, the idea has spread abroad that vaccination is a preventive, but it is erroneous. All the phenomena of distemper are traceable to an altered condition of the blood, and Semmer of Dorpat, who has investigated the disorder on modern methods, comes to the conclusion that that fluid contains a special bacterium of the micrococcus form. When the blood becomes contaminated with the distemper poison almost every tissue in the body may become the seat of asthenic manifestations, and according as the symptoms are most intense in any one system of organs has the disease been considered to assume a special type, such as the hepatic, pulmonary, intestinal, cerebro-spinal, or catarrhal. It is not evident to what the occurrence of either of these types in any particular case is traceable, but it is remarkable that when the disease is prevailing in an epizootic form some one special type markedly predominates. Certain conditions of the system seem to favour the development of the disorder, which in this respect resembles strangles of the horse; thus the young are especially liable to suffer, but it may occur in animals of any age; also it is especially frequent among foreign animals, more particularly those recently imported, and it is most severe in type and symptoms in animals which are subjected to specially artificial systems of management. Various defective sanitary conditions, such as damp, ill-drained kennels, too low feeding, want of light and fresh air, and no exercise, have been considered to generate it spontaneously, but this view must be received with the greatest caution. Such influences certainly render animals liable to attack, but the contagium of the disease is so wide spread, and its communicable nature so little recognised among people in charge of dogs, that we ought to hesitate before considering this specific disorder as capable of originating spontaneously. It is well worthy of inquiry whether in everyday practice there are not several distinct disorders diagnosed roughly as "distemper," every attack with typhoid symptoms being deemed an instance of the affection. Doubtless variola is sometimes thus confused, and, also, those remarkable malnutritions which are caused in the dog by deficient light and defective feeding, and which manifest themselves as ulcerative degeneration of the cornea and of the bowels are usually considered to be distemper.

Symptoms.—The poison after incubating in the system for a period estimated as varying from one to three weeks induces febrile disturbance. As a rule the local manifestations are those of nasal catarrh; they begin by a watery discharge from the nostrils, which becomes mucous and subsequently purulent and most tenacious, gluing the nasal alæ together, and obstructing the respiratory passages. The eyes simultaneously are involved in the catarrh, and quickly become the seat of a muco-purulent discharge which glues together the eyelids, so that in the morning they cannot be separated without artificial assistance. Changes in the blood supply of the Schneiderian and conjunctival membranes lead ultimately to ulceration as a result of defective nutrition; thus in time the nasal discharge may smell most foul and be occasionally intermingled with blood; the eye-changes consist in the appearance of one or more opaque spots which increase in size and extend inwards, sometimes they produce complete perforation with escape of the aqueous humour. In other instances abscesses form in the substance of the cornea and burst; they are surrounded by a ring of congested blood-vessels, but evacuation of their contents is followed by rapid clearing and thorough repair. Ulcerative changes are, in bad cases, found affecting the mucous membrane of the mouth, especially the gums against the teeth, the mouth is laden with sordes and smells most foully. This ulceration may extend to the lips, face, and neck in very severe cases (Blaine). Cleanliness of mouth, eyes, or nostrils materially lessens their liability to ulceration. During the progress of these symptoms the dog is out of spirits, listless in movements, and falls away most rapidly in flesh; he endeavours to keep in a warm place and away from observation, and in the earlier stages may vomit freely, and usually is troubled by a husky cough. Distemper is a disease the *prognosis* of which is attended with a very great deal of uncertainty; sometimes the anæmia " pulls the animal down " to such an extent as to make it seem probable that he will be utterly unable to survive the attack, and yet he suddenly takes a turn for the better, and improves with the greatest rapidity. Not rarely in the earlier stages of the disorder he suddenly seems to improve, his fever is less, his membranes clear up, and he seems to be progressing most favorably until convulsive twitchings, or deficient power in the hind limbs, or extreme excitability indicate the imminence of the nervous system becoming involved, either in the form of epileptic fits, chorea, or paralysis. It is noted that especially dogs of fancy breeds and high nervous temperament are liable to epileptic fits when suffering from distemper; the least excitement, even an angry word to another dog, will sometimes bring on this complication. In the earlier stages these fits, especially when they are not recurrent and paroxysmal, are looked upon as not a bad sign, but when they occur in more advanced cases and rapidly succeed one another, the patient is generally ultimately killed by them. In their phenomena and manifestations the epilepsy, chorea, and paralysis differ little from those affections when they are due to other causes. The paralysis is generally paraplegia and usually precedes the fatal result. More rarely the symptoms shown in these nervous cases are those indicative of brain pressure, and the patient may walk round in one direction continuously in a state of stupor for some time.

Young dogs suffer most from the *intestinal form*, which seems determined by irritation from the presence of worms in the bowels, or, perhaps, reflexly by teething. There is generally in the disorder a tendency to looseness of the bowels, and the evacuations, at first laden with mucus, are liable to become dark coloured and of most foul odour. When blood begins to appear it indicates ulceration of the bowels and the case is desperate. Colicky pains are not unfrequently present, and after death a very considerable portion of the bowel may be found spasmodically contracted.

In the *respiratory form* of the disease the symptoms are those of bronchitis of an extremely asthenic type, and corresponding lesions are found post mortem, in addition to those indicative of general derangement of the blood.

In the *hepatic form* there is severe jaundice, with its ordinary indications, and the depression of the system is most extreme.

Skin eruption, varying from puncta to large purulent accumulations beneath the cuticle, sometimes occurs. Far from constituting a favorable critical evacuation, it is generally considered to indicate the imminence of fatal termination to the case. In India it has seemed to me much less ominous, and skin eruption is frequently followed by recovery, the blebs burst and repair rapidly ensues, the skin remaining scurfy for some time. The most frequent seat of this eruption is over the belly.

Semmer of Dorpat records as present on *post-mortem examination* the following appearances :—Body emaciated, eyes and nostrils glued with purulent mucus. Lungs reddish brown, heavy, dense in consistency, and having their parenchyma infiltrated with fibrinous exudate. Commencing cell-infiltration of the alveoli, respiratory mucous membrane reddened, tumefied, and covered with mucus (or muco-pus). Brain and spinal cord œdematous (and their membranes highly congested and the seat of serous effusions in some cases). Liver bright yellow and of nutmeg-like appearance, and studded with brick-red and brownish-red streaks and spots, these appearances being due to fatty degeneration. Spleen enlarged and with a marrow-like infiltrate. Kidneys congested and fatty, but this state (as also the granular degeneration of the liver) not constant. The digestive and urinary mucous membranes present stellate patches of hyperæmia and ecchymoses. Muscular tissue of heart pale, and commencing to undergo fatty degeneration. Blood watery, serum contains many "globular bacteria," isolated or in ball-like clusters, or adherent to both red and white corpuscles. Also, in addition, some delicate and fine staff-shaped bacteria. The liver-cells and tubuli uriniferi full of bacteria. The urine brownish red and muddy, containing red and white corpuscles and epithelial cells, and many bacteria of both kinds, either free or enclosed in the blood-corpuscles or in the cells. Twenty-four hours after death the bacteria were very numerous, but they disappeared when putrefaction commenced. In the earlier stages the lungs are found in a state of œdema, later they show the signs of broncho-pneumonia ('Deut. Zeit. f. Thier-med.,' Band i, p. 204). In addition to the above, ulceration or infiltration of the nasal membrane and of that of the intestines, especially the ileum, and affecting particularly the solitary glands and Peyer's patches, congestion and dropsy of the pericardium, swelling of the lymphatic glands, especially those of the mesentery, and engorgement of the gall-bladder with thick bile have been noted. Spots due to ecchymosis are very frequent on the different serous membranes.

Treatment comprises prevention and cure. We must respect the opinion, almost universally entertained, that the disease arises spontaneously, but at the same time we must adopt every measure of disinfection and isolation necessary to prevent contagion. Semmer relates a remarkable case where the disease was conveyed to two puppies from the carcass of an animal which had been left in the cold for fourteen days prior to examination, a most extraordinary instance of contagion, which some will be inclined to consider rather one of spontaneity. However that may be, there can be no doubt that hitherto disinfection has been too much neglected in this disease. Of course thorough disinfection involves destruction of carcasses, dressings, &c. We must avoid being imposed on by vaccination or inoculation as preventives. We must insist on careful avoidance of contact with the sick, especially in spring and autumn, and with young dogs. Some dogs are capable of resisting contagion, but very few escape the disease altogether, and it may recur several times. Improved kennel hygiene should be insisted on when distemper is prevalent, and it may be necessary to "cross" a breed which seems to specially suffer from this disorder, and thus to an extent counteract any hereditary liability to it. When neglected, or in very hot weather, distemper assumes what Blaine has termed the *virulent or putrid type*, in which considerable ulceration of mucous membranes of the mouth, nostrils, and rectum takes place, the evacuations are most foul, and the body is coated with offensive discharge. The duration of attacks of this disease ranges up to three weeks, and during the whole of this time the tendency to extreme debility is most marked, and our principal resource in *medicinal treatment* lies in supporting the strength of the patient in every possible way. We know no specific remedy for this disorder, but medicines will be of value in dealing with the complications which occur; thus the catarrhs, eye lesions, epilepsy, chorea, jaundice, diarrhœa, and so on, will be dealt with on the principles elsewhere detailed in this work, but we must studiously avoid all debilitating influences and measures. Laxatives, blisters, and bleeding have been recommended, but should be never resorted to; even the mild preliminary emetic which is spoken of as "sometimes cutting short a threatened attack" must be administered only in the very earliest stages and with excessive caution. The effects of setons may be tried for chorea when a sequela of distemper, but not during its active stages. Worms should be expelled from the alimentary canal as soon as possible, because they are apt to induce intestinal or epileptic complications. While in every respect careful nursing is being carried out, especially cleanliness being insisted on, the animal should receive quinine in port wine or in beef tea or mutton broth. Strong coffee is considered of special value in arresting the tissue changes so apt to occur in this disorder, and some of the salts of iron, such as the carbonate and the citrate, may be resorted to for a gentle tonic action. Nunn uses three to five grains of sulphate of quinine in a little dry sherry as a tonic for small dogs, or liquor arsenicalis five drops twice a day. It is remarkable to what an extent the animal may be reduced before death occurs and with recovery still possible. No disease of the dog requires more sustained and careful treatment and nursing than distemper, and in none is more fully exemplified the maxim that "while there is life there is hope." The vegetable tonics should be persisted in throughout the attack. Once the animal takes a turn for the better he will be found to improve very rapiply.

DIPHTHERIA of the dog and the horse have been dealt with by Principal Robertson, then of Kelso, in the 'Veterinary Journal' for 1875, p. 82. He found it extremely fatal, only three or four recoveries having occurred in between twenty and thirty seizures. The outbreak was in a kennel of high-bred greyhounds; it first appeared among the puppies, and nearly all of them died before any of the older dogs were affected. The kennel-man thought the disease was distemper. The average duration of cases was a little over two days, but it always, when fatal, proved so before the fourth. The structural alterations were confined to the fauces and air-passages anterior to the glottis; the glands of the throat and neck, however, were swollen, and the urine was opaque, increased in density, and charged with albumen. The disorder was observed in three types: in the *first* there was high fever from the outset, acute local inflammation, the mucous membrane of the fauces being dark red, tense, glistening, and smooth (apparently in consequence of infiltration of its submucous tissue). All the gland structures of the mouth and throat were more or less swollen or tender, so that deglutition was almost impossible. Emesis and diarrhœa were sometimes present. These symptoms were succeeded by a second stage, in which there was marked depression. The characteristic grey exudation appeared only when the animal survived over twenty-four hours; it was arranged in stripes or spots, always adherent, glossy, tenacious, soft, and devoid of structure, varying in thickness in different situations. *Type number two* was less acute, the fever less marked, and the local lesions never severe enough to entirely prevent deglutition. The glands of the throat and neck were early swollen, and increased in size rapidly. Owing to extensive infiltration of the areolar tissue there was very awkward carriage of the head, and the patient was very restless until coma set in. The *third type* was nasal. With less fever than in the other forms the animal was dull, had sore-throat, and a sanious discharge from the nostrils and from the mouth (the latter mixed with saliva). In these, death supervened less rapidly than in cases of the other types, and before death the mouth became laden with sordes, the breath fœtid, and the lymphatic glands much swollen. Autopsy showed that the disease had involved the posterior nares but that the pharynx was most affected. Of the animals which recovered one was temporarily blind of both eyes from opacity of the cornea, another suffered from clonic spasms of the face and neck followed by paraplegia, but ultimately thoroughly recovered. The outbreak occurred in kennels in a very unsanitary state. Law mentions " croup " as one of the diseases of the dog and recommends its treatment by emetics. Bossi records a case where a dog ate excreta from a child with diphtheria, and died on the third day from suffocation. Autopsy showed the mucous membrane of the fauces pulpy and denuded of epithelium. Membranous exudation was here and there found, forming compact, thick, adherent excrescences, or ulcerations blackish and very deep. The inflammation extended to the pharynx and larynx. The heart and lungs were blackish and flabby, and contained pitchlike blood, and several fibro-albuminous concretions. Letzerich, in ' Virchow's Archiv ' for April, 1875, p. 178, describes how a dog was vaccinated with matter to which a small amount of diphtheritic material had been added. On the third day after, a soft swelling was observed at the seat of inoculation. The wound became indurated, gaping, and covered with a whitish, doughy-looking exudate. The swelling continued until the dog died, when wandering vegetable organisms were found in the various organs. Local diphtheria had occurred followed by secondary general diphtheria ('Veterinary Journal,' 1875).

Eczema Epizootica is transmissible to the dog, and cases are recorded in which it has resulted from consumption of milk of affected animals. Veterinary Surgeon D. C. Pallin related a serious case in a cat in which the palate was much disorganised, and which originated in this way.

Relapsing Fever, "Surra," has been conveyed by inoculation to dogs. The spiral organisms found in the blood in that affection propagate their species, and are

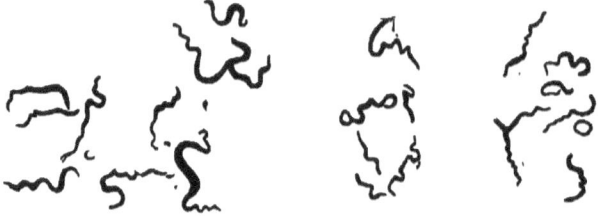

Fig. 22.—Surra organisms, "Spirilloids."

very active in the blood of the dog. The period of incubation is about ten days, the relapsing character of the fever is well marked, and at length the animal dies from exhaustion.

Anthrax, although not very frequent in carnivora, yet is seen in the dog more often than is generally supposed. It is liable to result when dogs have access to the evacuations of cattle affected with the intestinal form of anthrax, also from consumption of uncooked flesh of animals which have succumbed to either of the varieties of this formidable disorder. Perhaps the form most frequently assumed by anthrax in the dog is the intestinal, in which the animal suffers colicky pains; the evacuations from the bowels are mixed with blood; sanguineous matter may be expelled from the stomach by vomition, convulsions ensue after a period of deep depression, and the animal speedily dies. It is remarked that recovery takes place more frequently in the dog than in herbivora, and, moreover, that more of the former escape after exposure to infection than of the latter. However, occasionally the incautious use of a diseased carcass as food gives rise to severe disease and high fatality in a whole pack. In the most severe cases the animal falls dead, and no marked lesions are found after death, but the blood is black and thick, and the spleen enlarged. Generally some blood extravasations and petechiæ of the serous and mucous membranes are present, and yellow gelatinous material is thrown out round the lymphatic glands, especially those of the mesentery. Rougieux gives an interesting account of an outbreak among foxhounds near Paris, which is quoted *in extenso* in Fleming's 'Veterinary Sanitary Science and Police.' The disease began as swelling of the parotid (lymphatic ?) glands ; then a tumour, small and round, occurred on some part of the head, rarely on the body or limbs. Soon acute œdema of the tissues around the tumour set in, and respiration was so interfered with as to threaten suffocation. The skin covering the tumour and the buccal mucous membrane became ecchymosed and gangrenous, viscid saliva flowed from the mouth, the fæces were mixed with blood. The disease lasted seldom beyond five days, and death or improvement was noted about the third day. We need not enter into details as to the anthrax contagium and so on, for the veterinary surgeon will apply his knowledge as gained from experience of the disease in herbivora. Toussaint ('Veterinary Journal,' xi, p. 150) reports the results of experiments with his system of *anthrax vaccination* as applied to the dog. He finds that young dogs from birth to six months old readily contract the disease from simple puncture, and die with the blood laden with bacteridia, local and gland lesions being well marked. The first inoculation causes slight fever, and in two cases he found slight œdema at the seat of inoculation. All four animals vaccinated resisted successive inoculations by puncture. It is noteworthy that in the dog authrax is very liable, when it does occur, to assume the form of blebs or pustules in the mouth (which are probably the lesions described by Blaine as being by "country people" attributed to the animal having killed a toad or serpent, or having been poisoned with some acrid herb), and dogs affected with anthrax have been known to convey the disease by their bite.

VARIOLA is rare in the dog and apt to be confused, in hasty diagnosis, with the cutaneous form of distemper. There seems to be a form of variola special to the canine species, but evidence tends to show that smallpox and vaccinia are communicable to the dog, the former being liable to prove fatal, and the effects of vaccination being usually trivial. Bösenroth ('Mag. f. Thierh.,' 1860, p. 341) shows that Var. caninæ is communicable to man. Canine variola very closely resembles the allied disorders in man and the sheep; indeed, Leblanc has recorded an instance of where eleven out of seventeen dogs died as a result of disease caused by ingestion, as food, of the carcasses of sheep affected with sheep-pox. The variola of the dog is *malignant* or *benign;* the pox may be confluent or discrete, it passes through the various stages of erythema, nodule, vesica, and pustule, and the latter becomes flat or even concave on the surface. Desquamation follows and brownish spots are left. As these disappear, small hairless spots with scars or "pits" are left to indicate the seat occupied by the pox. These eruptions occur especially where the skin is thin, such as over the belly, inside the forearms and thighs. Their advent is preceded by fever, they cease to develope as soon as the desquamative stage has set in for any of the pustules. There are cases in which the respiratory organs are involved, and bronchopneumonia, with specially early and rapid pus formation from the whole of the lining mucous membrane of the airpassages, occurs, there being much mucous râle and profuse discharge of pus from the nostrils, cough in the earlier stages, and later very stertorous breathing, and a tendency to rapid fatality. In other instances the alimentary mucous membrane is invaded, there being profuse diarrhœa of dark, offensive, bilious evacuations. In all cases the breath and skin excretions smell very foul. The disease specially affects young dogs (under eighteen months old), and very young animals almost always succumb to the fever and prostration present, especially as in young animals the disease passes through its several phases most rapidly.

Treatment consists in careful nursing of the patient, disinfection, isolation, and, when necessary, stimulants, vegetable tonics, and febrifuges. It is stated that in case of recovery the animal is free from future attacks ; a property of disease which has received the technical name of "*unicity.*" Heat is said to favour eruption and confluence of the vesicles, whereas cold checks the eruption, and undue exposure is almost sure to prove fatal to an affected animal.

GLANDERS is communicable to the dog. Lafosse mentions a case where the animal became affected through living in a stable with a glandered horse; Polli induced the disease in dogs by intravenous injection of disease matter and spreading it on wounds; Renault conveyed it to dogs by inoculation from horses, and reinoculated horses from these dogs successfully ; one third of the dogs inoculated took the disease ; the infected dogs lived from three and a half to five months. Hertwig failed to cause true glanders by feeding dogs on the flesh of glandered horses, although Nordström succeeded. St. Cyr found the induced disease seldom fatal except when caused by intravenous injection, and he remarks that probably one attack ensures future immunity, but this has not yet been established. Chancres seldom appear on the nasal membrane in the dog ; in Nordström's cases there was bloody discharge from the nostrils, œdema of the head, redness of the eyes, and death, although generally spontaneous cure follows.

MEASLES.—In 1876 a case was related before the Epidemiological Society where a dog (which four years before suffered from distemper) licked the hand of a child suffering from severe measles. In twelve days' time the animal sickened, a nasal discharge appeared on the second day, and on the fourth day it died with marked congestion of the throat and air-passages ('Veterinary Journal,' iii, p. 226).

CHOLERA has been supposed communicable to and by

dogs. In this connection Surgeon-Major Fairweather's report on the cat epizootic at Delhi is worthy of notice. The disease occurred during the prevalence of cholera, and cats were dying by scores, sometimes after a few hours' sickness with vomiting and profuse purging. The post-mortem appearances were like those of cholera. All the cats had a pinched appearance, eyes sunken in their sockets, and the viscera seemed to occupy less space than usual. The intestines generally contained nothing but thin fluid like rice water, in one or two instances slightly tinged pink, always completely free from bile. Congestion of the tube in one or two cases but no ulceration. Liver generally flabby, gall-bladder full. Kidneys much congested, lungs shrunken ; heart, a loose black clot on the right side. An attempt to convey disease by cohabitation with a diseased animal failed, as also did ingestion of the intestinal contents. Human choleraic evacuations given to cats caused vomition and purging, and in some cases death, with the ordinary appearances of the cat disease. Subsequent experiments did not confirm this result ('Veterinary Journal,' iii, p. 209).

TUBERCULOSIS.—There certainly occur in the dog some disorders of the lungs, mesenteric glands, and other parts of the body which have all the appearance of tuberculosis, and yet we are not aware of any distinct evidence having been brought forward that true "consumption," due to the tubercular bacillus, is ever found in the dog. Observations made by MM. Colin and Laulanié tend to prove the occurrence in the dog of certain false tuberculoses in the lungs due to the filaria or strongyles in the lungs (Colin) or the arrested ova of *Strongylus vasorum* (Laulanié). The latter observer shows that the adult strongyles live in the right ventricle and the larger divisions of the pulmonary artery, and from there the fecundated ova pass into the pulmonary arterioles and capillaries, where they are hatched, and the embryos soon migrate into the smallest bronchi, where they are found in great numbers in sections of lung tissue examined under the microscope. The lungs in which these parasites reside are studded with small, grey, semi-transparent granules, which realise all the appearances of granular phthisis, but they accumulate towards the base of the pulmonary lobes and become more and more rare towards the apices, the reverse being the case in true phthisis. "The ova or embryos arrested in the fine arterioles become the starting-point of a *nodular arteritis, combining in its structure all the characters which, since the days of Koester, have been assigned to the elementary follicles of tuberculosis. There is found, in fact, in the centre of each nodular mass an ovum or an embryo embedded in a giant-cell.* The latter is surrounded by a more or less abundant circle of epithelial cells, as well as an external embryonic zone, which frequently tends to become fibrous." In fact the ova or embryos have given rise to just such lesions as would be presented in a true tubercle the result of the bacillus of Koch; detection of the latter in a nodule is the only exact method of diagnosis of tubercle. In dogs we find nodular disease, developed in some puppies, acquired in others, which stunts their growth and keeps them in an unthrifty, emaciated state. This is especially found as a hereditary derangement in very small terriers, pugs, and other toy breeds which are bred to the smallest possible size to suit the fancy of purchasers. Breeding in and in is supposed to be a special influence at work to induce nutritive derangements in such cases. The hereditary and congenital tendency to disease is liable to be excited by want of exercise and sufficient food, use of contaminated or bad milk, damp dwellings, and exposure to cold. In some cases the little wizened pup seems to "run all to belly," and to be preternaturally sharp, and with a pinched expression; his coat is harsh, mucous membranes pallid, bowels irregular; he suffers much from thirst, and his nose is often dry and hot. Post-mortem examination will show a *tabid* state of the mesenteric glands; an enlarged, indurated condition by which they are rendered quite unfit to bring about the changes in the chyle necessary to render it nutritious. In other cases cough, fœtid breath, liability to disturbances in respiration, and a tendency to diarrhœa are present, and lung disorder is found after death.

Strict hygiene, tonics (such as cod-liver oil and iron iodide), good food, warm bed, and, especially, carefully arranged, easily digestible diet, may keep the patient alive for some time, but as he is quite unfit to breed from and will require constantly the most careful attention, it is generally better to destroy a pup thus affected. Messrs. Gowing have recorded a case in the 'Veterinarian' for 1868 in which the liver was dark in colour and speckled here and there with yellow granules. These were so numerous as to render the gland almost globular in shape, compact in texture, and of the consistency of an ordinary fatty tumour; its section was granular and mottled with minute, yellow specks. The heart was fatty; a fellow pup died of the same disease, marasmus, with distended abdomen due to tuberculous deposit.

SEPTICÆMIA.—It is a remarkable fact that although it is, to an extent, natural for dogs to feed on putrid material, yet when decomposing matter enters a wound fever of a typhoid character, followed by collapse and speedy death, occurs; or occasionally the animal recovers after profuse diarrhœa with most offensive evacuations. This accident is especially liable to occur in bitches in which laceration of the lining membrane of the genitals has occurred and the fœtus is in a decomposed state. The fever sets in some eighteen or twenty hours after inoculation. After death the tissues in general are found œdematous and spotted, and it will be observed that they undergo speedy decomposition. Treatment comprises stimulant tonics internally and the use of antiseptic and disinfectant lotions in frequent washing out of the diseased parts. The disease in relation to parturition is carefully described in Fleming's 'Veterinary Obstetrics.'

NON-SPECIFIC DISORDERS OF THE BLOOD.

RHEUMATISM is somewhat frequently seen in dogs, especially those used for sporting purposes, and generally due to the neglect of an old sporting rule to "lie warm and dry." Thus it is seen most often in damp kennels, with a cold, north-easterly aspect, and where the beds are too near the ground, especially if such kennels be ill-ventilated and kept in a dirty state. The disorder is most frequent in spring and also occurs frequently in autumn. Mayhew considers it one of the diseases which result from over-feeding. It assumes either the acute or the chronic form; the latter often results from an attack acute at the outset. The frequency of rheumatism in its several forms among canine patients contrasts rather remarkably with its infrequence in herbivora. Dr. Richardson's experiment on the artificial production of rheumatism has a great deal of interest to the canine pathologist. A solution of lactic acid was thrown into the peritoneal sac of a healthy dog, which died in two days, and on post-mortem examination showed marked endocarditis; there being tumefaction of the tricuspid valve; an inflamed and enlarged condition of the aortic valves, with fibrinous beads along their edges; endocardium red; pericardium dry (Watson). These cardiac lesions are seen also in the naturally acquired rheumatism of the dog, in which animal, however, the disease is remarkable for its little tendency to metastasis and for the frequency with which it affects the bowels, causing either inflammation or torpor of them, as specially noticed by Blaine. Also there is less liability for the joints of the limbs to be affected than in man, and more frequently there is paralysis as a sequela, which may be temporary or permanent. The most frequent forms of rheumatism in the dog are *lumbago* and " *chest founder* " or " *kennel-lameness.*" The former is denoted by arched back, tenderness of the loins, the animal moves as if half paralysed behind and is most averse to move. He screams pitifully when touched. Generally fever at first runs high and the belly is hot and painful on pressure. The bowels are very liable to be constipated, and, until they can be acted on, the fever and lameness will not yield to treatment. *Chest founder* is rheumatism affecting the subscapular muscles and those which unite the fore extremity to the trunk, so that the animal suffers pain when the shoulders and the fore limbs are manipulated, also the dog moves about stiffly and with difficulty as though somewhat paralysed before. Youatt speaks of *kennel-lameness* as due to washing hounds, and, with Nimrod, he " deprecates even their access to water in the evening after hunting." He speaks of the disease as an ill-understood affection, and seems to distinguish between it and chest founder. The latter he mentions as a " singular complaint, and often a pest in kennels which are built in low situations, and where bad management prevails ; where the huntsman or whippers-in are too often in a hurry to get home, and turn their dogs into the kennel panting and hot ; where the beds are not far enough from the floor, or the building, if it should be in a sufficiently elevated situation, has yet a northern aspect and is unsheltered from the blast, chest founder prevails." He considers it sprain and inflammation of the subscapular muscles from long-continued and considerable exertion, leading occasionally to paralysis, as specially seen in pointers.

Treatment of rheumatism consists in opening the bowels, and then giving salicylic acid, colchicum, or iodide of potassium, together with alkaline carbonates. These substances may be tried in turn, or, since the disease is very liable to recur, at the several attacks. Local treatment should comprise warm water applications followed by stimulating liniments to the affected parts. In chronic cases the joints are liable to become affected and most painful in cold weather ; setons or blisters may then prove useful. The diet must in all cases of rheumatism be moderate and carefully regulated, and the patient be kept in a warm, dry place, under strict hygienic conditions. With a view to prevention, excessive washing must be avoided, and, especially, leaving the animal to dry when he has been washed. In cases of incipient or partial paralysis the effects of acupuncture or electricity may be tried.

RICKETS is a disease of special interest to the canine surgeon, for, of all domesticated animals, the dog is most liable to it. MM. Voit have carefully studied the relations of this disorder to the use of food devoid of calcareous matter. They found that "young animals, with imperfectly formed skeletons, suffer more from deprivation of lime than adults and directly in proportion to their size. Young dogs fed exclusively on fat and flesh became extensively rachitic without any other modification of the general nutrition. The disease consisted in an inflammation of the parts of the bones in which growth occurs, and especially in the most freely moveable rays of the limbs. A similar process occurs, even though the aliment contains sufficient lime, when, from any cause, such as disturbance of digestion or use of too great quantities of principles tending to

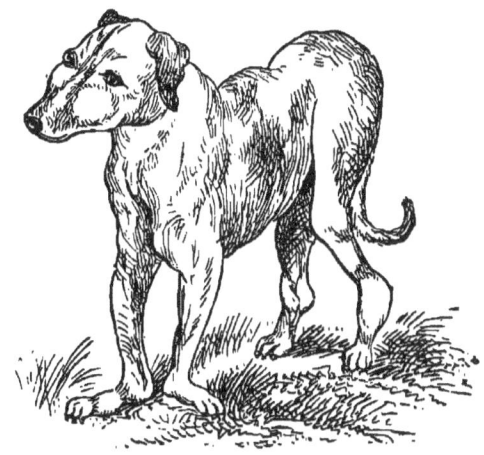

FIG. 23.—Rachitic dog (HILL).

increase the amount of excrement, a small proportion only of the lime in the food is absorbed." These facts agree closely with the conclusions of practical observers that the disease depends on improper food, indifferent ventilation, and the want of exercise, which is so essential to the efficient action of the bowels and development of the frame. It has been observed, also, that it prevails as a hereditary disorder, especially among pugs and small bulldogs (Blaine), and the breed of wry-legged terriers is supposed to have had its origin in the effects of this disease. Hill very justly warns us against concluding that all animals in which the legs are twisted and deformed are suffering from this disorder, for young dogs which have not been allowed sufficient exercise during development will have bodies too heavy for their legs, and the latter will yield under the superincumbent weight and, moreover, will, like all imperfectly used parts, develop but indifferently. Also green-stick fractures of the limb bones, and bones not "set" straight in young animals, give rise to deformity of the limbs. In truly rickety animals the joints especially will be found enlarged, and the head and belly will be disproportionately big. The disease appears at birth, the bones are soft and yield under the weight of the animal, also it is observed that only false union results from the frequent fractures in such cases. The nutritive functions in general are unsatisfactory in natural rickets, and it has been supposed to result especially from the deleterious practice of breeding in and in.

Treatment.—Avoid rickety parents or such as have produced rickety offspring; rear all pups on correct hygienic principles, giving good food, healthy milk, plenty of exercise, and adequate shelter. Give bone dust, lime-water, crushed egg-shells, with a view to supplying calcareous matter to the system, and especially give such nutritive diet as is found to be best suited to the digestion of the patient. Cod-liver oil has been proved to be highly beneficial.

LEUKÆMIA, as a disease of lower animals, has been specially studied by Siedamgrotzsky. It consists in excess of white corpuscles and relative deficiency of red, due to hyperplasia of the blood-making organs, spleen, lymphatic glands, and marrow; hence it assumes three forms, *splenic, lymphatic,* and *myelitic,* as discoverable by autopsy rather than diagnosis. It is more frequent in dogs and cats than in other domesticated animals, and a predisposition to it is most marked in middle and advanced life. The cause is obscure; the spleen is most frequently enlarged, the result of prolonged hyperæmia of the organ, which at first is soft and distended with blood, later, firm and anæmic, its margins become rounded and its surface rough from thickening of its capsule. The Malpighian corpuscles may be enlarged to the size of a pea. The lymphatic glands and medulla undergo similar hypertrophies in other cases, and lymphoid tissue may be developed in other parts of the body such as the liver and kidneys. Leukæmia is best diagnosed by observation of the blood from the living animal. After a progressive anæmia, extending over from three weeks to five months, the patient dies. No therapeutic method has yet been pointed out likely to affect a cure. Innorenza, of the Naples Veterinary School, has described this fatal disorder as a sequela of distemper.*

JAUNDICE or ICTERUS is bile-poisoning of the blood ; a condition of frequent occurrence in the dog, especially as a symptom of liver disorder. It is found in hepatitis, obstruction of the bile-ducts by inspissated gall or by calculi, in the earlier stages of malignant liver disease, and especially in gastro-duodenal congestion, where the tumid condition of the mucous membrane prevents the free pouring of bile into the bowel. Occasionally it results independently of *appreciable* disorder either of liver or alimentary canal, where the activity of the bile-secreting elements has become torpid after over-fatigue, sudden chills, exposure, or injury of the dog. Animals which have received over-doses of emetic and purgative medicine suffer from it, as also watchdogs constantly tied up. " In-whelp bitches occasionally become jaundiced from uterine pressure, which generally disappears after parturition" (Hill). This disease is known to sporting men and kennel men as "*the yellows.*" It is found in its most acute form in sporting dogs, especially greyhounds, whereas it appears in fancy breeds only as a primary stage in liver degeneration, or as an important symptom in intestinal disorders such as intussusception of the bowels. Constipation has been spoken of as a common cause, but it would be more correct to consider the two conditions simultaneous results of torpidity of the liver and want of exercise or suitable food. The abuse of emetics and purgatives gives rise to jaundice through the turges-

* 'Veterinary Journal,' iv, p. 60.

cence of the gastroduodenal mucous membrane which they produce.

Symptoms.—The animal is at first dull, sleepy, and disturbed in his sleep, thirsty, and refuses his food, and expels it when taken, by vomition. Bilious diarrhœa as indicated by dark stools is not unfrequently present, and some slight colic and pain on pressure over the liver may indicate a congestion of that organ. Soon the patient becomes feverish, but the attack is paroxysmal, much worse sometimes than at others. The skin becomes yellow and either dry and harsh, or else, as Mayhew accurately expresses it, "rather like a skin which had been well dressed by a furrier than one which was still on a living animal." The mucous membranes, too, are yellow and may become intensely so, and the urine in severe cases becomes so dark as to look almost red, and be commonly described as "bloody." The bowels now become very torpid, and the small amount of fæces expelled is of light brown or whitish colour. In the later stages the alvine evacuations are mixed with blood because the mucous membrane of the bowel becomes ulcerated. The patient at this stage is much "tucked up" in the flank, and the whole of the belly feels hard and tender; the dog is much reduced in flesh, his coat becomes rough, his gait staggering, and death follows, generally preceded by convulsions.

Treatment comprises careful nursing with administration of light soups and mucilaginous vegetable mixtures, which latter are especially useful for sheathing the ulcerated or congested gastro-intestinal mucous membrane from the acrid bile poured into the canal in the early stages. Small doses of sulphate of soda or sulphate of magnesia also assist to free the bowel from acrid bile; starch and laudanum enemata are sometimes required. The kidneys may be gently acted on by nitre in small doses; quinine and magnesia also are of benefit. When the fever runs high a small amount of blood may be extracted and the sweet spirits of nitre given as a febrifuge and sudorific. Fresh, cool, dry air and gentle exercise are most valuable as curative means and to prevent recurrence.

DISEASES OF THE BLOOD. 71

ANÆMIA in canine patients sometimes assumes a marked character and can be only imperfectly explained. Thus, dogs kept in dark places, ill cared for, badly fed, and totally deprived of exercise, undergo nutritive defects in almost every tissue of the body such as are particularly visible to the observer in the cornea, which becomes opaque in spots and ulcerated, as in rabies occasionally and in distemper not rarely. Hæmorrhage or chronic disease may give rise to a similar state, as denoted by extreme weakness, pallor of visible membranes and skin, bleeding imperfectly when cut, coldness of the mouth and extremities, and, finally, paralysis and death. Autopsy shows a general bloodlessness of the tissues and a tendency to serous effusion, such as may have set in, under the form of anasarca of perinæum, intermaxillary space, or limbs, before death. The animal, weakened by disorder or maltreatment, may be subject to fits before death occurs. Tonics, stimulants, good nutritive food, and strict hygiene, with determination and removal of the cause operative in the special case, is the line of treatment suited to anæmia Where it is associated with a liability to fatty degenerations of organs, as denoted by weak heart with a tendency to palpitation, the effects of small doses of chlorate of potash long continued may be tried.

PLETHORA, although common in dogs, is not liable to give rise to pathological states primarily, although secondarily it causes considerable disorder of almost every part of the body. Mayhew alludes to its occurrence, in the form called " *Foul,*" among sporting dogs which are, in spite of close confinement and cessation of work at the end of the season, still highly fed as though in full work. Under such mismanagement the dog soon suffers from a very serious complication of disorders, each of which requires its special treatment.

FEVER in the dog is almost always sympathetic or one of the symptoms of blood disease, but there are, nevertheless, cases in which while fever runs high no local disorder can be detected. Malarious influences undoubtedly affect the dog, inducing recurrent fever with absence of appreciable lesions detectable post mortem, a few petechiæ on the lungs and beneath the endocardium, a slight excess of serum in the serous sacs, a general pallor of the tissues, and a tendency to congestion of the small bowels only being present. Such cases supervene on severe exertion and exposure. They obstinately resist varied forms of treatment, and much light has yet to be thrown on their nature.

The system of the dog is specially liable to nutritive changes. Thus fatty degenerations and tumours, as well as a tendency to extreme obesity with age, are extremely common, and has been noticed in spaniels, especially among the different breeds. We shall see how the occurrence of fatty degeneration of the heart and liver is frequent in toy terriers and other pets.

CHAPTER IV.—DISEASES OF THE CIRCULATORY SYSTEM.

INTRODUCTION.—There is a simplicity about the circulatory apparatus of the dog which renders it but little liable to disease; indeed, the works on Canine Pathology of two well-known authors have no notice of this important system of organs. Doubtless with increasing knowledge of the subject we shall gradually learn that cardiac diseases of an organic form are most frequent in sporting dogs; those of a functional nature in toy breeds. The *heart* is thin walled and almost globular in form; the apex is directed backwards, and the right side lies against the upper surface of the sternum; but, as the breast bone is inclined obliquely downwards and backwards, the difference in the position of the heart between carnivora and herbivora is not great. The apex is rounded and formed by *both* ventricles, and the two sides are fairly equal in size. The pericardium is posteriorly attached to the tendinous portion of the diaphragm. The arterial and venous systems are capacious and well developed, but the lymphatic apparatus is small in proportion, although the receptaculum chyli is large and runs far forwards in the chest. The relative development of blood and lymph systems as above explained is quite in accordance with the sanguine temperament of the animal. It is estimated that the heart of the dog may vary from ·3 to ·7 per cent. of the weight of the animal.

FIBROUS DEPOSITS ON THE VALVES OF THE HEART result from rheumatism. They form a rough surface on which fibrin becomes deposited before death, and the clot may prove fatal by occluding the cardiac openings or entanglement of the valves in such a way as to interfere with their

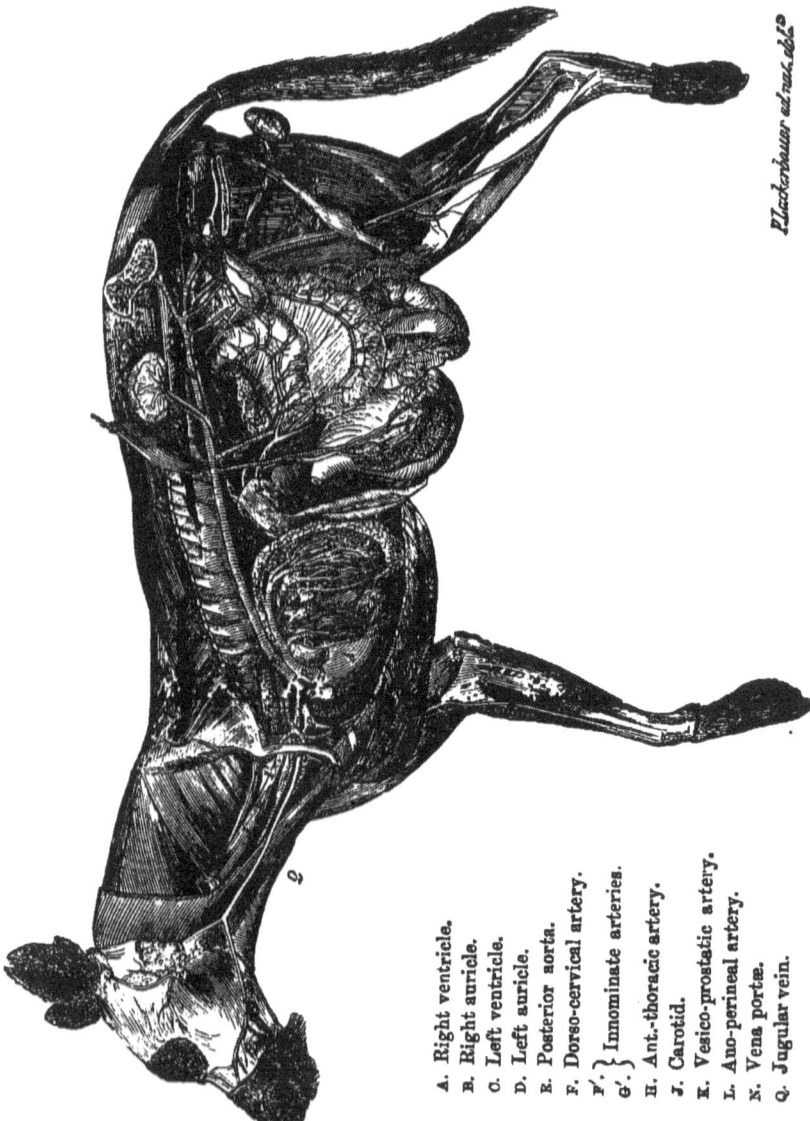

FIG. 24.—General representation of circulatory organs of the dog (CHAUVEAU).

A. Right ventricle.
B. Right auricle.
C. Left ventricle.
D. Left auricle.
E. Posterior aorta.
F. Dorso-cervical artery.
F'. G'. } Innominate arteries.
H. Ant.-thoracic artery.
J. Carotid.
K. Vesico-prostatic artery.
L. Ano-perineal artery.
N. Vena portæ.
Q. Jugular vein.

DISEASES OF THE CIRCULATORY SYSTEM. 75

action. Nothing can be done to remedy this state of affairs; indeed, it is not often diagnosed, but when a patient liable to rheumatism has irregularity of the pulse and a sharp jerky beat of the heart, also a rushing sound is detectable on auscultation, this condition may be suspected. It has further been observed that animals suffering in this way are liable to give a sudden shrill cry and fall in an attack of syncope. Small doses of calomel alternated with iodide of potassium are indicated; quiet must be enforced. But the animal is at any time liable to drop down dead.

FATTY DEGENERATION OF THE HEART is frequent in pampered asthmatical pets. It must not be confounded with fatty deposit in or upon the heart, for it is much more

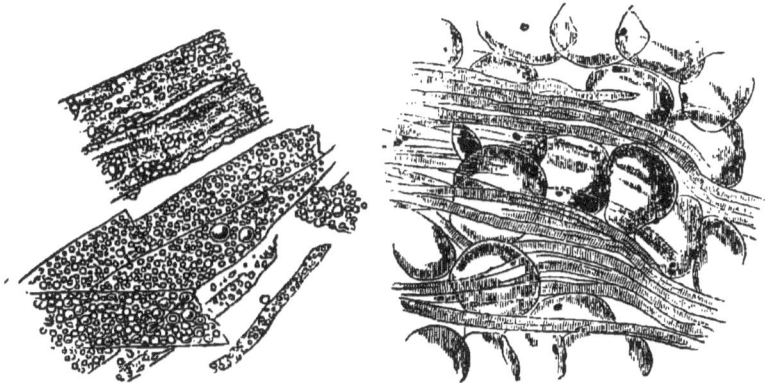

FIG. 25.—Fatty degeneration (QUAIN).   FIG. 26.—Fatty infiltration (QUAIN).

serious, being a true degeneration of the muscular fibres of the organ. There is a marked want of tone in the pulse and heart's beat in these cases, and an incapacity for even moderate exertion, but there are no infallibly diagnostic symptoms; death ensues from syncope. Post mortem the heart is found to be pale, soft, and greasy on section.

RUPTURE OF THE HEART is occasionally seen, but not so frequently as in the horse and other working animals. Youatt reports a case in which the animal suffered from valvular disease, as denoted by the symptoms already described and verified post mortem, and died suddenly from a giving way of the wall of the left ventricle. The rent was some two inches in length, and at the base of the ventricle where the walls were thin. There was evidently concentric hypertrophy of the cavities. Youatt calls attention to this case as remarkable because the *left* ventricle had given way, whereas in man and most quadrupeds the right is the one which generally is ruptured. A mild excitement, playing with another dog, was the immediate cause of death. This indicates the necessity for the avoidance of unnecessary excitement, whether from exercise or emotion, when we suspect heart disease. A nutritious laxative diet and small doses of tonics may assist in prolonging the animal's life in cases of heart disease, but unless he is a "pet" or pensioner it is not advisable to keep him as a valetudinarian.

DISEASES OF THE PERICARDIUM generally result from those of the pleura. An accumulation of serum in the sac sometimes occurs, and may be suspected when the heart's beat is very feeble and the sounds obscured. Generally the animal dies suddenly. But disorders of the pericardium are rare in the dog. Delafond records a successful case of *punctured wound of the pericardium and walls of the chest.*

HÆMATOZOA, CANINE.—In 1878 Dr. Patrick Manson contributed to the 'Chinese Customs Gazette' (*vide* 'Veterinary Journal,' vol. vi) a most interesting article on Chinese Hæmatozoa. He describes two forms, *Filaria immitis* (v. *Canis cordis*) and *F. sanguinolenta.*

Filaria immitis, a familiar cause of sudden death among English dogs imported into China, is commonly known as "WORM IN THE HEART." It is estimated that two out of every three dogs in China are hosts of this parasite, as may be determined by microscopical examination of a few drops of blood from a living animal. The embryo worms will be seen moving freely in a serpentine manner. These cause apparently no inconvenience to the host, but the parent worms "are found coiled up in the right ventricle of the heart for the most part, sometimes extending through the tricuspid valve into the auricle and even into the superior vena cava, and very generally through the semilunar valves far into the pulmonary artery and its branches." In one case forty-one worms were counted. They are found massed together in a thick bundle, consisting of the larger female and the male, which has a long narrow tail curved like a corkscrew. The smallest female measured was seven inches in length. How the parasite enters the circulation has not been ascertained. The position in which the mature parasite is found (in the *right* rather than left side of the heart) is fortunate, for only the immature embryos, smaller than a blood-corpuscle, can escape the filtering action of the lungs, whereas unhatched ova or *débris* resulting from death of the parasite, if they passed into the smallest arteries, would give rise to emboli. Probably tuberculoid disease results occasionally from such bodies becoming entangled in the lungs.* The most frequent ill effect, however, is an interference with the valves of the heart and the capacity of the pulmonary arteries and its branches; it is nevertheless astonishing how large the rope of worms may be without causing death. It is noticeable that death generally results after exertion, such as fighting, when the energetic action of the ventricle may force one or more worms suddenly into the pulmonary artery, or entangle them among the valves. After a day or two, during which there are indications of breathlessness or of failing circulation, death may come on suddenly. Hollingham mentions dulness, constipation, absence of fever, frequent vomition, irregularity of the pulse, and frequent "fits" as the symptoms in a case observed by him ('Veterinary Journal,' vol. xiii).

* Rivolta, when at Turin, was surprised to find embryos of *F. immitis* in the blood of dogs which had during life presented all the symptoms of dumb rabies, and which, from a clinical point of view, might be regarded as suffering from that disease. He attributes the symptoms to the embolic action of the embryos (1875). He also believes they may cause death by producing pulmonary congestion, or enterorrhagia, or grave hæmorrhagic typhus ('Veterinary Journal,' June, 1882).

Filaria sanguinolenta (Schneider and Lewis) has been found by Dr. Lewis in the œsophagus, thoracic aorta, and neighbouring parts of the pariah dogs of Calcutta. Schneider found it (or a closely allied form) in the walls of the stomach. Dr. Manson has found it in Amoy and considers that all dogs there which have attained any considerable age are or have been its host. It is debated whether the embryonic filariæ in the blood are of this form or of *F. immitis;* the latter view is most probable, and Rivolta says that when embryos are found in the blood the mature *F. immitis* can always be found in some part or other of the body. There are no absolutely diagnostic symptoms of their presence during life. " On opening the thorax of an affected animal and drawing the heart and left lung over to the right side, the straight part of the thoracic aorta may be seen studded with small tumours, ranging in size from a small pea to a bean, and the anterior and lateral surfaces of the œsophagus bulged out by tumours perhaps as large as a walnut, and where several of these are in juxtaposition a large lobulated tumour may conceal the œsophagus altogether. To the touch these tumours are hard, though at points there may be a feeling of deep fluctuation. If the aorta is excised and split open, its inner surface is found, at the points corresponding to the tumours on the outside, to be more or less deeply sacculated, the inner coat roughened and the outer coats thickened. In the latter worms at different stages of development may be found, or perhaps the sacculation and external bulging may only be evidence that a worm has once been there, but has disappeared. When the worm has reached a certain stage in its development a minute orifice can be seen on the inner surface of the tumour, communicating with the cavity containing the animal. Through this hole a purulent fluid can be expressed; this on microscopic examination is found to be loaded with characteristic ova, and cells resembling those of ordinary pus. The tumours in the œsophagus occupy the muscular wall, and generally are much larger than those of the aorta. On the inner surface of the œsophagus a small hole is, as a rule, to be seen, perhaps several, communicating with the cavity of the tumour, and through this the purulent egg-laden fluid can be easily expressed; sometimes, and by no means rarely, part of the mature filaria protrudes through this hole and hangs loose in the channel. I have found, connected with the œsophagus, mature tumours embedded, as I have just described, in the muscular walls, similar tumours cretified and enclosing fragments of a long dead filaria, small pedunculated tumours of filarian origin projecting into the channel, and long tunnels burrowing between the coats, in some part of which a parasite can be found. In addition to these, the more frequent situations, the animal may be found in large or small glandular-looking lumps in the areolar tissue of the posterior mediastinum, or encysted between the costal and pulmonary pleura. In all these situations I have found them, and also in the same dog. When small, the parasite is found alone, closely invested by the peculiar tissue it seems to create around itself, lying as it were in a tunnel; but when mature it is found loose in a large tumour, in company with one or more (eighteen I found in one instance), all encapsuled in a common and perhaps cretified cyst, and floating in a purulent fluid." Dr. Manson surmises that the embryo when swallowed attaches itself to the œsophagus, pierces the walls of this tube, remaining in them and becoming encysted, or penetrating farther to the thoracic aorta. Small worms are most often found in this latter situation, in which probably they do not generally attain maturity, deserting it for the more favorable situation in the œsophagus. Immature worms are single and lie closely invested in their tunnels; the mature are always in company, sometimes in considerable numbers, and float loose in a fluid enclosed in a cyst. From this it is inferred that when the worm becomes sexually mature it migrates in search of one of the opposite sex. There are such points of difference between the two blood-worms of the dog as prove that they are not members of the same species in different stages of development, as their frequent occurrence in the same host might lead us to anticipate. We continue to quote from Manson's paper:

"I believe there are three serious morbid conditions produced by *Filaria sanguinolenta* :

"1. *Stricture of the œsophagus*, more or less complete. This most frequently occurs when several large tumours are formed, especially when they are grouped together near the cardiac end of the tube, the most frequent locality. Regurgitation of food and slow starvation will be the consequence, unless the tumours diminish in size by the escape of their contents or death of the filariæ.

"2. *Pleurisy.*—This is not uncommon in dogs here, and, I think, is often caused by the bursting into the pleura of a tumour which does not find vent for its contents by opening in the usual way into the œsophagus or aorta. I have found very distinct evidence of this occurrence in one instance. In it worms were found crawling about amongst recent adhesions in the serous cavity.

"3. *Paralysis of the hind legs.*—This is also common here, and is, I believe, caused by plugging of the capillaries of the spinal cord by ova escaping into the aorta. The brain is not affected, as the filaria tumours are seldom, if ever, situated on the cardiac side of the arteries proceeding to the head. Other affections are doubtless produced by the ova in the intestine, kidneys, and other viscera, but I have no knowledge of them or information to offer on this very interesting and important point."

In the blood of man (in about 8 per cent. individuals in Amoy) a filaria is found, and may possibly be a cause of stricture of the œsophagus. There are some important anatomical differences between the human and canine hæmatozoon.

It is commonly supposed in China that dogs get worms in the heart from drinking the water of stagnant pools about the settlement, and worms in all respects resembling *Fil. immitis* have been found in rain water. After attaining a length of about three and a half inches they disappear, and the water becomes putrid and swarms with embryonic filariæ. It is possible that the embryos of the filaria are obtained ordinarily from human fæces.

Simpson records, in the 'Journal of Anatomy and Physiology' for May, 1875, an interesting congenital malformation in the dog—*persistence of two pre-caval veins*, owing to Cuvier's left duct remaining pervious.

At a recent meeting of the Pathological Society of London, Mr. Harrison Cripps mentioned that he had seen aneurysm in hounds, and that the celebrated greyhound Master McGrath died from aneurysm of the aorta.

Apart from the pathological conditions already noticed as affecting the circulatory apparatus of the dog, doubtless there are others which, as being less frequent and less marked, have not yet been recorded. They do not need special notice from us here since their diagnosis, prognosis, and treatment must be based on general surgical and medical principles.

CHAPTER V.—DISEASES OF THE RESPIRATORY SYSTEM.

INTRODUCTION.—In accordance with the large size of the circulatory apparatus and the activity of most of the vital processes in the dog, we find the lungs and air passages well developed. We have also reason to believe that in all the carnivora the lungs are very active organs of excretion. High development and great functional activity entail frequent disease of parts, and so we find that the dog is very liable to derangements of the respiratory organs. But it is to be remarked that, in accordance with the mode of life, disorders of the lungs range themselves in two classes, the *acute inflammatory*, to which greyhounds and other dogs of speed are liable, and the *degenerative*, which attack the pampered pets of the boudoir. To these may be added a third class, *parasitic*, our knowledge of which is due to the researches of Dr. Osler of Montreal, Laulanié of Toulouse, and Rivolta of Turin. We are not aware of it having been recorded as occurring in England, but it seems frequent in the south of Europe.

OF THE NASAL CHAMBERS AND THEIR ACCESSORIES.— *Anatomy and Physiology.*—The anterior nostrils are guarded by moveable boundaries the basis of which is a complex cartilage which is very thin and flexible. The skin of this part of the body is thick, highly glandular, free from hair, and in health is moist and cool. A more or less marked channel runs from the centre down to the upper lip. The nasal chambers are small, but vary much in relative development in the different breeds; their turbinated bones are small but complex; the ethmoid cells, on the contrary, are very well developed and complicated. The sinuses are very small, being practically limited to a frontal cavity. It must be remembered that the mouth is the main passage for air expired or inspired in the dog. In the emergencies of respiratory disease and extreme exertion it is kept open and the tongue protruded; the velum pendulum palati is short and so allows free respiration through the mouth. Indeed, for respiratory purposes we must consider that the nasal passages have only an everyday function; they become quite subordinate in emergencies. They are, in some breeds, however, very important organs of smell, but from a respiratory point of view will bear no comparison with the wide, complex, highly vascular, air-warming passages seen in herbivora. This adaptation of the mouth to passage of air as well as food is possible in carnivora, because in them the food is rapidly passed through the mouth and feeding takes a very short time, whereas the mouth of herbivora is generally filled with food and its passage occluded in the act of mastication or remastication. These details are necessary in order that we may understand why diseases of the nostrils and their accessories are of so little importance and so infrequent in the dog as compared with the horse.

CATARRH or CORYZA, which is congestion, running on to inflammation, of the lining membrane of the nasal chambers, is somewhat frequent. It results from exposure to draughts, severe weather, east winds, and especially when the dog has been used to warm, close quarters.

The *symptoms* are fever, more or less severe, discharge from the nostrils, at first watery, later mucous, and then becoming intermingled with pus. The animal snorts out the discharge frequently and snuffles in breathing. The eyes generally water through sympathy or the excess of tears flows through the *ductus ad nasum;* persistent sneezing and an occasional cough are present. The disease is liable to extend and involve the pharynx and larynx. When the sinuses are invaded the animal is very dull and "snuffles" a good deal. Difficulty in swallowing and tingeing of the nasal discharge with the liquids of the food, also severe cough, show that the throat is becoming involved.

As *treatment* simple nursing generally suffices, but in

severe cases the animal's head must be held over steam frequently during the day, and stimulant tonic medicine administered with care—say a drachm each of nitrous ether and tincture of gentian, to which may be added a grain of ipecacuanha or of squills; to be repeated every eight hours. The strength must be sustained by nutritious diet of a laxative character; neither emetics nor cathartics should be used. When the disease persists tonic pills may be given.

When SORE-THROAT sets in, great care must be taken in administration of medicine; in severe cases nutritive and tonic enemata must be resorted to. The throat should be bathed freely and the mouth and nostrils steamed. There will be some swelling of the neighbouring glands, cough (often very troublesome), difficulty in swallowing, breathing somewhat obstructed, return of liquids through the nostrils, a fetid state of the saliva which trickles from the mouth, breath offensive, voice altered or lost. In these cases our main aim must be to support the strength of the patient. When the swelling is very great it may be necessary to perform tracheotomy. In sore-throat the parts should be carefully examined through the mouth in order that we may assure ourselves of the absence of sharp pieces of bone (firmly fixed on the top of the molars, for instance) or other impediments to free passage. This disease must not be mistaken for "dumb madness," in which the mouth cannot be closed, and there is no cough.

OZÆNA bears the same relation to coryza as dysentery does to diarrhœa. In it the mucous membrane is chronically inflamed, perhaps ulcerated, the turbinal structures may be diseased, and pus or vomited matters may be so entangled in them as to keep up the irritation and be unable to escape.

The *symptoms* are chronic snuffling and a rattling sound in passage of the air through the chambers; dulness; a discharge of ichorous or sanguineous pus from the nostrils often smelling very fetid. It is generally seen in small-faced dogs such as pugs and bulldogs. Youatt considers it a disease of old age which must take its course, although in extreme distress an emetic may be required to give the animal relief, and the passages must be kept as clean as possible. He continues, "I scarcely ever knew a very old pug that had not it to a greater or less degree." Syringing the passages with solution of zinc chloride or permanganate of potash lessens the smell and promotes cure.

PARASITIC OZÆNA is of frequent occurrence, for an arachnidan, *Pentastoma tænioides,* takes up its abode in and near the nasal chambers of the dog. It is the mature

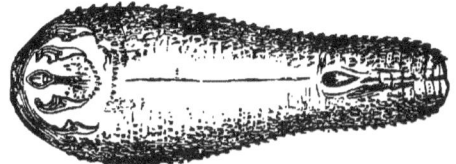

FIG. 27.—Pentastome (COBBOLD).

form of *Penta. denticulatum,* which infests the abdominal viscera of horses, ruminants, man, and other animals, and is tolerably frequent in various parts of Europe. "Our dogs commonly obtain the worm by frequenting butchers' stalls and slaughter houses, where portions of the fresh viscera are apt to be inconsiderately flung to hungry animals" (Cobbold). Professor Dick records a case of sudden death, supposed to be the result of poisoning, in which three pentastomes had wandered into the larynx, trachea, and left bronchus respectively, probably in search of warmth, and so suffocated the animal ('Veterinarian,' 1840, p. 42).

As these parasites are formidably armed and rough, they cause a good deal of irritation when they are migrating from one part of the nasal chamber to another. The patient rolls violently, sometimes in a convulsive fit, rubs the nose with his paws or against the ground, sneezes paroxysmally, champs the jaws, and occasionally death ensues. These active movements result from the parasite being disturbed in some way, as by cold, frosty air. The pentastome is said to take twelve months in development, and during this time the host suffers from coryza, and, in the event of death, the effects of long-standing inflammation of the Schneiderian membrane will be found on post-mortem examination.

Treatment comprises inhalations of chlorine, chloroform, or tobacco smoke, also various injections into the nostrils, and trephining.

POLYPUS IN THE NOSTRIL is a tumour of mucous membrane with more or less fibrous tissue; it hangs into the nasal cavity and may be visible from the exterior or extend back into the pharynx. It gives rise to slight ozæna and to stertorous breathing. Occasionally there is some bleeding in full stream from the nostrils. When possible it must be removed by ligature or excision. Gohier records two cases detected by resistance to the passage of a gum sound. Gourdon says, "Pass a thread by means of a Belloc's sound on one side of the tumour through the pharynx and into the mouth; then passing the sound to the other side of the tumour draw out the thread through the nostril and saw away the rest of the polypus with a concealed saw."

Snorting is sometimes a habit, but often it indicates a low form of congestion of the lining membrane of the nostrils, in which case astringent injections may remove it.

EPISTAXIS, bleeding from the nostrils, occasionally occurs in plethoric dogs during hot weather, and especially in tropical countries; it may also result from a blow on the head. Cold water applications and quietude will soon cause it to cease.

OF THE LARYNX, TRACHEA, AND BRONCHI: DISEASES OF THE AIR PASSAGES.—In anatomical conformation these parts present nothing of special importance as bearing on pathology and surgery. The cartilages are well developed, and very liable to undergo calcareous change; each tracheal ring has its extremities widely apart superiorly. The passages in general are wide open and well developed to admit the free entry and exit of air.

COUGH, which is generally an indication of disease

DISEASES OF THE RESPIRATORY SYSTEM. 87

of the lungs, pleuræ, or air passages, or due to gastric, intestinal, or other abdominal irritation, occasionally occurs independently of any apparent local disorder, and so assumes a primary pathological importance. Although it is a matter of doubt in every such case whether there is not some reflex irritation at work, there are certainly some instances in which previous disease or general atony of the system leads to a relaxed state of the blood-vessels of the laryngeal mucous membrane and chronic cough in consequence. This must generally be regarded as a sequela of laryngitis. It occurs most often among pampered animals, especially when made to run about or moved into the open air. They cough violently and spasmodically, with a harsh, grating sound, ejecting froth and mucus from the mouth. The paroxysms only occur when some special cause of irritation is at work, and, although the symptoms are something like those of "bone in the throat," there is no impediment to the air or food passages recognisable, and fits of coughing come on. These cases are often of considerable duration. The pathological state of the laryngeal mucous membrane persists and can be only counteracted by tonics and strict attention to regular exercise and feeding. Expectorants prove temporarily useful, and hydrocyanic acid in doses of a half to one drop is much recommended.

LOSS OF THE VOICE, partial or complete, results temporarily from violent prolonged barking.* The chordæ vocales become relaxed and congested, and require rest before they can resume their functions. It is common among small excitable dogs at shows, but after the excitement is over, if the animal be kept quiet, the voice will be restored.

Snoring is another result of a relaxed state of the structures of the throat; it depends on want of tone of the velum palati, and sometimes constitutes a very serious objection, as in pet dogs which sleep in their fair mistress's bed-chamber. It results from pampering, and

* Hill says, "I have also observed what may be designated a temporary or simple form of laryngitis in sheep dogs when gathering flocks together."

may often be removed by reduced diet, increased exercise, and tonics.

ACUTE LARYNGITIS is much less frequent in the dog than the horse, and its effects are, in the case of most breeds, of less importance. It occurs as a distinct disease, but is most frequently a part of the state known as angina or sore-throat. Fever runs high, there is a certain amount of coryza, pressure on the throat at once causes a painful hacking cough, the voice is either lost or very hoarse, and the respiratory efforts are frequent. Snorting has been remarked as one of the earliest indications. Whether the disease be due to exposure, direct injury, or extension of inflammation, it requires active treatment, because it is most distressing and debilitating, and is very liable either to chronically disorganise the laryngeal lining membrane or to extend down the windpipe and involve the bronchi and lungs in the inflammation. Serous effusion beneath the laryngeal mucous membrane, ulceration, or chronic congestion are liable to remain after the subsidence of more acute symptoms. The painful and distressing condition known as *laryngismus stridulus* has been seen in the dog. It is denoted by the sudden occurrence of extreme difficulty in breathing, and a crowing sound with each respiratory act. It seems to depend on reflex spasm of the laryngeal muscles.

Treatment of acute laryngitis although active must not be heroic. It is a mistake to administer violent emetics and cathartics—indeed, in bad cases the irritability of the throat renders it difficult to administer any medicine whatever. In the acute stage the animal must be carefully housed, kept in a warm, moist atmosphere, allowed to inhale steam, and, where there is much distress, a little chloroform. The throat should be freely fomented and a stimulating lotion rubbed in, and enemata of milk or broth with solution of belladonna extract should be given.*

---

* Harms injected 0·07 grammes of hydrochlorate of morphia in solution subcutaneously in a dog with dry laryngeal cough of four weeks' standing. Narcotism for two hours followed, but the animal gradually regained sensibility, and in two and a half days left the hospital all right.

Occasionally it may be necessary to perform tracheotomy. A little tempting liquid food ought to be placed before the animal and frequently changed, even although untouched.

In *chronic* cases tonics are beneficial, in fact the treatment above suggested for cases of chronic cough must be tried, together with the application of blisters or other stimulants to the throat, or a seton may be inserted. Mayhew warns us that "the jugular veins in this animal are connected by several large branches, which run just where the seton would be introduced. These could not be pierced with impunity, nor ought the seton to be left in so long as might induce sloughing, when the vessels probably would be opened; for, as the dog badly sustains the loss of blood, the result would surely be fatal." He also says, " I found great improvement result from wearing a very wide bandage, which was kept wet and covered with oil silk, round the neck."

OF THE ESSENTIAL ORGANS OF RESPIRATION.—The chest of the dog is capacious, and highly expansile. The diaphragm has but a small central tendon. The anterior opening into the chest is much smaller than in the horse (relatively). The left lung well overlaps the heart by its middle lobe, a fact to be remembered in auscultation. The pulmonary tissue is delicate but firm, and the air sacs are large in proportion. The posterior mediastinum is so stout as to suffice to prevent mechanical passage of serous accumulation in the chest from one pleural sac to another. The total amount of bone entering into formation of the walls of the dog's chest is very small; his ribs are rounded and not numerous; their cartilages of elongation are well developed and rounded; the bones of the sternum are numerous, rounded, long, and narrow. The muscles of respiration are all much more fleshy than those of herbivora, and the fore limbs may be freely moved backwards and forwards. The dog, too, is more freely manipulable for auscultatory purposes than larger animals, accordingly the conditions are very favorable to the adoption of *auscultation* as a means of diagnosis of his diseases. The lung-sounds can be freely heard in almost every part, and although they differ slightly in tone from those of the larger animals, will prove diagnostic. Direct auscultation or stethoscopic may be made; I always prefer the former.

Percussion, succussion, and *measurement* may assist the diagnosis, but we must mainly depend on auscultation to guide us in diseases of the chest.

INFLAMMATION OF THE ORGANS IN THE CHEST is generally complex—bronchi, lung tissue, and pleura being all more or less involved—but the main seat of disease varies in different cases, and generally we find that the structure which is first invaded is most severely affected. It is convenient to consider the three principal forms of chest inflammation together, because they exhibit a number of similarities in causes, symptoms, and treatment, and practically we have to deal with them as a whole. Thus a dog is brought to us in a state of fever, panting hard, with a cough and shivering fits. We first inquire into the *cause.* He may have been exposed to cold, whether by not being properly dried after a bath or a swim, by not being well clothed on removal of his coat in cold weather, by accidental exposure through a cold night, by being taken out on a cold day without his rug on, in the case of toy pets, or imperfect housing. So far we have nothing to specially guide us, but if he has been treated for catarrh or laryngitis for a short time, we probably have bronchitis in the main to deal with, or if he has had a kick or wound in the side, the case is one of pleurisy.* Some of the *symptoms,* too, will further our diagnosis. Thus, in bronchitis the breathing is very quick but even, and not apparently painful; in pneumonitis it is quick and oppressed, and in pleurisy the expiration is prolonged and the inspiration sharp and jerky. Auscultation shows the mucous râle throughout the chest as soon as bronchitis

* Pure pneumonia is the most frequent cause of mortality among the larger felines imported into Europe. It has been noticed that even a very small amount of lung consolidation suffices to kill a tiger. In the 'Veterinary Journal,' viii, p. 169, is a most interesting record of a case of pneumonia in a tiger by Mr. L. Butters, M.R.C.V.S.

has well set in, earlier a sibilus is present. In pneumonia crepitus, dulness, and, later, various forms of râle and sibilus are present, either generally diffused or circumscribed. In pleurisy there is first friction-sound, later an absence of sound from the lower part of the chest according to the amount of serous fluid effused. The loss of sound alters with change in position of the patient, and the superior limit of dulness is sharply defined and alters from time to time in accordance with variations in the amount of effusion. Such, roughly, are the indications afforded by auscultation. It is unnecessary to enter further into detail here, because the information as to the exact extent of disease will depend entirely on the experience of the observer, and practically we find the different intrathoracic phenomena so intermingled that each case is a problem in itself and must be solved from its own indications. Cough is present in all cases, but that of bronchitis is moist and wheezy, that of pleurisy paroxysmal, painful, and cut short, and that of pneumonia occasional and small. In pleurisy there is pain on pressure of the sides, also twitching of the muscles of the walls of the chest. In both bronchitis and pneumonia the temperature of the expired air is increased, but especially so in the latter. The pulse is frequent, hard, and small in pleurisy, oppressed and fast in pneumonia, frequent but generally soft in bronchitis. In bronchitis and pneumonitis there is frothy (rusty or whitish) expectoration, but not in pleurisy. The dog with inflammation of the lungs and pleura sits up with his fore legs apart (*vide* Fig. 1, p. 9), often in the latter stages of the disease he stands until he falls down to die. It has been remarked that in pneumonitis the extremities become extremely cold, and the nose, instead of dry and hot, is cold and very moist. In the latter stages of chest disorder the patient becomes a pitiful object, much emaciated, struggling for breath, obstinately sitting or standing, tongue purple and hanging from the mouth and very foul, breath most offensive, teeth covered with sordes; a haggard and distressful look. When HYDROTHORAX has set in the animal lies down most unwillingly, œdematous swellings supervene, the breathing becomes very laboured, and the intercostal spaces dilated. " The beating of the heart will likewise afford a decided characteristic of the complaint; for the hand, placed on one side of the chest, will be affected with a kind of thrill, very different from the usual sensation presented by the beating of the heart of a healthy dog" (Blaine). In consequence of the frequency of pleurisy of only one side of the chest of the dog, cases of hydrothorax are generally much protracted in him. There is a similarity in the *treatment* of these disorders. The main principle to go on is to support the system in every possible way with a view to enable it to resist the ravages of disease, and to promote those changes which lead to cure. Whilst special stress must be laid upon careful nursing, it must not be forgotten that good cool air is a tonic and a necessary for existence. Emetics, bleeding, drastics, and other debilitants must be carefully avoided. Stimulants, febrifuges, with expectorants when the lungs and bronchi are most affected, must be freely given. Fomentations or stimulant applications to the sides are most beneficial. Later, tonics and absorbents, such as the iodide of iron, in two-grain doses, and more powerful stimulation to the sides is required, and in advanced pleurisy *paracentesis thoracis*, performed in the usual manner, has proved beneficial, the puncture being made between the seventh and eighth ribs and near the sternum. Bleeding has been recommended in the earliest stages of pneumonia, but is very risky practice, which we are not prepared to advocate, especially with Blaine's warning that "if it is performed after the second day the dog commonly dies under the operation." In all forms of inflammation of the chest it is admissible to regulate the bowels by mild doses of laxatives, saline or oleaginous.

VERMINOUS BRONCHITIS.—For our earliest information upon this most interesting form of disease as affecting dogs, we are indebted to Dr. Osler of the Montreal Veterinary College. He describes an outbreak among the pups at the kennels of the Montreal Hunt Club. The affection was con-

DISEASES OF THE RESPIRATORY SYSTEM. 93

fined almost exclusively to animals under eight months old ; it was pneumonic in nature, and had proved fatal in several

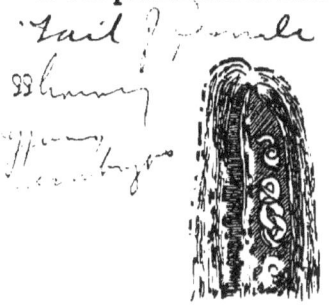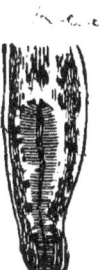

FIGS. 28, 29.—Parasites of verminous bronchitis. (From Hill on 'Dogs,' after OSLER.)

instances. Fifteen couples were attacked, and twenty-one animals were lost. Three of the couples were old dogs.

Symptoms.—" Among the initial symptoms disinclination for food and exercise, together with an unsteadiness of gait, amounting in some cases to a subparalytic condition of the hinder extremities, were the most evident. In fully half the cases convulsions occurred. There was rarely diarrhœa or any other symptom referable to gastro-intestinal disorder. Cough was not a prominent symptom, being absent in many of the cases ; when present it was short and husky, ' not,' as the keeper said, ' the regular distemper cough.' In the case brought to the infirmary the cough was well marked, and was dry and short. The pulse and respirations were increased and the temperature elevated. Towards the close all food was refused, and even, when fed, the soup was commonly vomited. Death took place in most instances quietly, though sometimes during a convulsion, and the keeper noticed that the pups which lasted the longest had the most fits. The duration of the disease ranged from three days to a week or even ten days." It showed itself during remarkably cold weather, and especially among young animals housed in a cold place.

Post-mortem examinations were made in eight cases, and

showed dirty brown frothy fluid in the passages, red consolidation of the lungs (only partial, however). "On slitting up the windpipe the mucous membrane is found covered with a dark frothy mucus. The membrane looks pale and natural to within an inch of the bifurcation, but at this point it becomes reddened, uneven from the projection of irregular little masses of a greyish yellow colour, which on close inspection are found to be localised swellings of the membrane, containing small parasitic worms, the white bodies of which can be seen lying upon, and partially embedded in, these elevations. They are most abundant just at the bifurcation, at the lower part of which several have emerged, forming an elevation three or four lines in height. About the orifices of the second divisions these little masses are also seen, and the whole mucous membrane of this region is deeply congested and somewhat swollen. Very few of the worms are found lying free on the mucous membrane; almost all of them are attached to the masses or buried in them. The smaller tubes, especially those leading to the diseased portions of the lungs, are filled with a dirty brown fluid, and on squeezing any portion of the organ quantities of it can be expelled. The bronchial glands are swollen." Each little elevation consisted of a nest of the parasites. Adult worms, free embryos, and ova were detected in mucus from the smaller tubes. The males were found to be smaller and less numerous than the females. No abnormality of the blood could be detected and no forms intermediate between the free embryos and the adult worms could be found. Osler terms the worm *Strongylus canis bronchialis;* the largest measure a quarter of an inch in length. He argues out the mode of invasion and supposes that the dried embryos are inhaled with the breath, and lighting on the mucous membrane find suitable conditions for their development. In two out of the eight bodies examined by him no parasites were found although pneumonia was present. But the phenomena of the enzooty seem to stamp it as truly parasitic, and naturally the youngest dogs, as having the least resisting power, were those which succumbed to the parasites. It is clear there is nothing diagnostic about the symptoms recorded, although possibly microscopical examination of expectorated matter would elucidate the cause of the pneumonic attack.

Treatment should be chlorine inhalations and stimulant tonics, such measures as are resorted to for cases of hoose in young cattle, an exact pathological equivalent of the disease under consideration. Therefore the intratracheal method of administration might be tried.

ASTHMA—CHRONIC BRONCHITIS—is, in the main, a disease of senility, and pathologically resembles the diseases of nostril and larynx already described as ozæna and chronic cough. Differences between these three diseases result from the structure and situation of the membrane involved. In each, however, atony is the primary element. The smaller bronchial tubes in the lungs have a well-developed muscular layer, which, with the mucous coat, becomes involved in true asthma and undergoes degenerative changes. The muscular tissue in the earliest stages is affected with spasm, and the mucous layer with chronic congestion. Later the mucous coat becomes thickened, and the fibres, often muscular, undergo fatty degeneration. The air passages become blocked up, and thus access of air to particular parts of the lung prevented; emphysema, true or false, then affects more or less of the rest of the lung. It is a mistake to draw a line, as some have done, between congestive and spasmodic asthma; both these conditions are present in all cases of the affection; at times the paroxysmal spasm proves so urgent as to mask the by no means less serious indications of congestion, and in others there is scarcely any indication of spasm. This disease is rarely fatal, although it causes extreme distress at times.

Causes.—Pets of fancy breeds, house and watch dogs, are most frequently the subjects of this disorder, because they have the fewest opportunities for exercise, they are generally highly fed, least inclined to exertion, and most liable to indigestion. Over-feeding, pampering in other ways, extreme obesity and want of sufficient exercise, are the principal causes. These begin to "tell" on animals as they grow old, but sometimes young animals become very asthmatical as a result of hereditary tendency.

Symptoms.—The earliest indications are those of indigestion, foulness of the mouth, flatulency, piles, frequent vomition, and a depraved appetite; generally there is a marked craving for flesh. Associated with these is a dry paroxysmal cough which is brought on by excitement, as when the animal is teased or made to take a short run. This cough proves very distressing and increases in severity; indeed, in some cases the distress is extreme, and the animal seems as if about to succumb to dyspnœa; marked shortness of breath follows every attempt to run, and generally some palpitation of the heart, for this latter organ in such cases is usually the seat of fatty degeneration or of extensive deposits of fat. When the paroxysms of coughing set in some frothy matter is expectorated and relief follows. The lung-sounds are variable and confused, the bowels generally constipated, and the general tone of the muscular system is low.

Treatment comprises (1) the adoption of measures to shorten the paroxysms and afford relief; such as inhalations of chloroform or amyl nitrite, small doses of prussic acid (Youatt), balsamic gums (Blaine), antimonial wine or ipecacuanha as expectorants, doses of narcotic agents as tobacco smoke, opium, or ether. Occasionally a stimulant to the walls of the chest affords immediate relief, or a hot bath is useful in cases of emergency. (2) The palliation of the want of tonicity in the system by strict attention to regular exercise, care of the coat, a vegetable diet limited in amount, and regulation of the digestive organs by occasional doses of aperients. (3) The avoidance of such causes as specially bring on spasms, as undue exertion and exposure to cold. Iodide of potassium or chlorate of potash in small doses long continued are said to be useful, and occasionally the desired effect results from a course of arsenic; vegetable tonics are of advantage as improving the digestion and the tone of the system in general.

In concluding our observations on diseases of the respira-

DISEASES OF THE RESPIRATORY SYSTEM. 97

tory organs of the dog, we may remark on *the rarity of acute pulmonary congestion and pulmonary apoplexy in this animal*, but that it does occur has been amply proved by Cadeac of Toulouse, who has published his researches in the 'Révue Vétérinaire.'

DISORDERS OF THE DIAPHRAGM seem not to have been observed in the dog.*

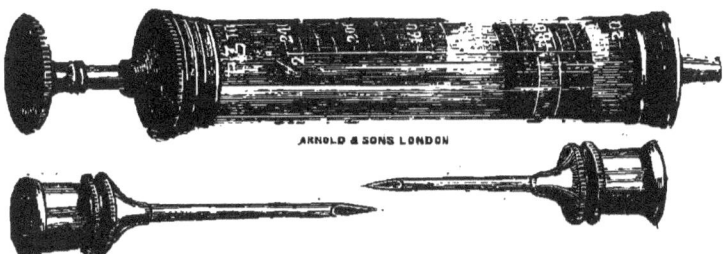

FIG. 30.—Patent syringe for intratracheal injection.

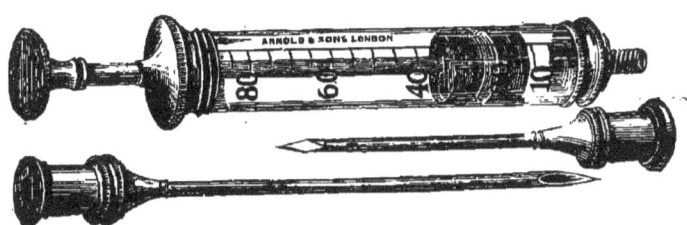

FIG. 31.—Improved patent hypodermic syringe.

* But in the 'Révue Vétérinaire' for August, 1886, Besnard, of Rochelle, gives a case of DIAPHRAGMATIC HERNIA of the dog. The whole intestine except the duodenum and rectum had passed into the chest through a rent in the fleshy part of the diaphragm, on the right side and high up. The greater part of the intestinal mass was contained in the omentum, which was, however, torn here and there. The lungs had in places become adherent to the bowels.

CHAPTER VI.—ON THE DISORDERS OF THE DIGESTIVE APPARATUS.

The Mouth and its appendages.—In carnivora the gape is wide and so the thin cheeks can, when the jaws are closed, be drawn out to form a pouch, which is used in place of a funnel for reception of liquid medicines. The lips are small and their muscles to an extent rudimentary; they are everted in some breeds by the long canine teeth, and are more or less papillated on their free margins. The palate is wide opposite the centre of the molar rows, but narrows in front; it presents imperfect transverse ridges. The tongue is thin and wide, often hangs freely from the mouth vibrating at its edges. It presents a central raphé, and in this is a remarkable fusiform mass apparently of cartilage. The operation of " WORMING," so frequently practised in days gone by, consisted in the removal of this organ by an incision into the frænum linguæ or else of the frænum itself. It was practised on young and mischievous puppies "to prevent their going mad." Its immediate effect was to prevent them from tearing carpets, rugs, and such like, with their teeth because of the soreness of their mouths thus mutilated. On this its reputation was based. It is cruelty, and any performance of this needless operation should be dealt with as such. The true physiological value of this extraordinary organ has not yet been demonstrated. The base of the tongue is wide and has numerous papillæ; the whole of the isthmus faucium is wide and capacious. We must notice the shortness of the pendulous palate as compared with that of the horse and its rudimentary uvula. Also, that the tonsils are well developed, being rounded, elongated from before backwards, and capable of receding into special

ON THE DISORDERS OF THE DIGESTIVE APPARATUS. 99

recesses during the passage of the food masses. It will be observed that the mouth is large and can open wide for purposes of prehension. The maxillary joint is so arranged as to admit only of up-and-down motion of the jaws; its interarticular cartilage is rudimentary. The muscles which close the mouth are stout and fleshy; everything points to the possibility of obtaining a firm, strong grip with the jaws, such as is essential to carnivora and the terror of burglars.

The TEETH are suited mainly for cutting. In the full mouth they are forty-two in number. Six small *incisors*, the

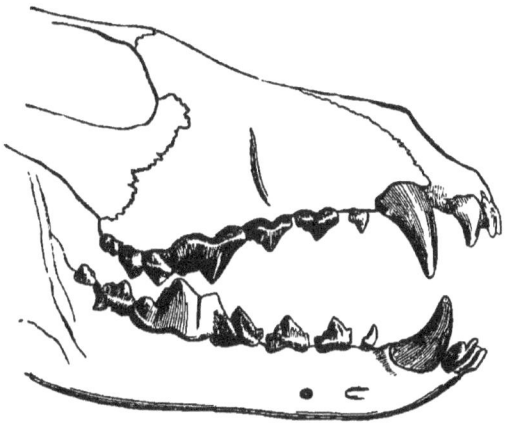

FIG. 32.—Dog's teeth (CHAUVEAU).

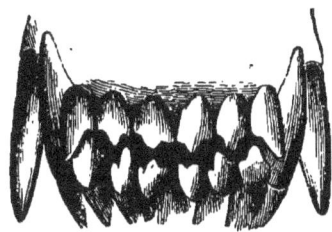

FIG. 33.—Dog's teeth (CHAUVEAU).

central of which are quite rudimentary and often lost early in life without any detriment to the animal; the laterals are a little larger and the corner ones almost tush-like, especially in the upper jaw. The four *tushes* are long, recurved, have large fangs, and so are formidable weapons of offence and defence, and useful for prehensile purposes. Of the *molars*, those anteriorly placed are rudimentary; especially the small premolars which are immediately behind the lower tushes. The fourth tooth in the upper jaw on each side and the fifth in the lower are the largest teeth, and they lose somewhat the sharp edge of the true canine molar and become widened. The teeth behind them are small and best adapted for crushing; but the back teeth are lost in the short-nosed breeds of dogs as the palate shortens with age, their fangs become exposed and carious, and the teeth actually drop out as functionally superfluous and structurally expelled for want of space. These molar teeth are not such ponderous, massive, complex organs as we see in herbivora, they are simple in structure, have but little crusta petrosa, and their fangs are numerous and small. We might think this simplicity of structure would secure them from such diseases as are seen in the horse, and undoubtedly it does so. The diseases of the teeth of the dog differ to a remarkable degree from those of herbivora. In the latter we find disorder due to overgrowth with non-apposition, in the former we find accumulations of tartar, loss of teeth, and caries, especially of the fangs.

TARTAR ACCUMULATIONS of a blackish colour are very frequently found on the teeth. They are greatest around the neck of the tooth and thus interfere with its proper fixture in its socket, cause ulceration of the gum, and absorption of the margin of the alveolar cavity. In these cases the mouth is very offensive to the smell, there is a certain amount of ptyalism, the lips may be ulcerated, and the teeth are loose. In some cases the teeth are even displaced by the amount of matter deposited. These unpleasancies are not often seen in healthy, hard-fed dogs, but prove very troublesome to pets, and a source of great disgust to their owners. They are caused by a vitiated state of the secretions of the mouth the result of indigestion, and secondly, the want of the natural means by which a dog's teeth are cleaned, namely, meals of meat large enough to require biting, and bone picking. If we throw parts out of use by our artificial methods of treatment they degenerate at once, and generally by that acute process known as disease. Of course old animals are most frequently affected in this way; it also seems that carious teeth are most liable to the deposit. The amount of fetid matter on these teeth should render us specially cautious in handling these animals, as a bite from them would be liable to take on unhealthy action.

Treatment comprises attention to the general health, removal of the tartar thoroughly with the instruments made use of ordinarily for scaling human teeth, washing the mouth out regularly and frequently with chloride of zinc lotion, made by mixing half an ounce of Burnett's fluid in a pint of water. Attention to any co-existing disorder of the teeth, and giving the dog a dish of bones to play with occasionally.

BROKEN TEETH are frequent in animals which learn to fetch and carry; *excessive wear* results from the same cause. When these defects are not extensive they cause little inconvenience, but in the case of old dogs allowance must be made and their food be duly prepared for them. Meat food requires but little mastication provided it be given in portions not too large for passage down the œsophagus. Sometimes what at first sight seems excessive wear is on closer examination found to be advanced caries.

DISPLACEMENT OF THE TEETH is the result either of accumulations of tartar or of persistence of the temporary teeth. The latter condition is most often seen in short faced, fancy breeds, which require some attention during the cutting of the second teeth. This trouble is seen especially with the tushes or fangs, which, after persisting for a time, become fixed to the bone and permanently retained, and filth accumulates between them and the permanent fangs, causing disease of the gum and bone and looseness of the permanent tooth. "To extract a temporary tush after it has reset is somewhat difficult and is not to be undertaken by every bungler. The gum must be deeply lanced; and a small scalpel made for the purpose answers better than the ordinary gum lancet. The instrument having been passed all round the neck of the tooth, the gum is with the forceps to be driven or pushed away, and the hold to be taken as high as possible; firm traction is then to be made, the hand of the operator being steadied by the thumb placed against the point of the permanent tush. As the temporary teeth are almost as brittle as glass, and as the animal invariably moves its head about endeavouring to escape, some care must be exercised to prevent the tooth being broken" (Mayhew). The molars of older animals may be displaced by tartar. If a loosened tooth is diseased it should at once be removed, but otherwise when cleaned it may become again firmly fixed in the jaw; of course this cannot be anticipated in very old animals. The teeth of the dog are easy of removal, whether artificially or accidentally, because they do not mutually support each other as those of herbivora, nor have they such large fangs deeply embedded in the jaw.

Cutting the tushes is an operation which is sometimes necessary; with puppies, to prevent them tearing things, when it is done simply by a pinch with bone forceps; or in older animals when unusually fierce, or if they have been exposed to rabies inoculation, to reduce their power of doing harm; in them the process of rasping is generally resorted to. Loss of the incisors is of little importance and not likely to interfere with the tenacity of the animal's grip; indeed, in those breeds where the under-shot condition of the lower jaw is natural, early displacement and loss of the incisors is to be anticipated as a physiological process. The non-occurrence, in so far as we are aware, of dentigerous cysts and superfluous, irregularly-placed molars in the dog, is probably due to the comparative simplicity in structure of his molars; and to the same cause we must also attribute the infrequency of hollow molars from caries of the crown.

CARIES of the teeth of the dog generally involves the fangs, and is the result of hereditary taint, excessive salivation, or indigestion from excessive and erroneous feeding. The symptoms in these cases are sometimes very urgent; extreme fetor of the mouth and breath, looseness of teeth with pain on pressure, deposits of tartar, and absolute refusal of food. *Treatment* comprises extraction by means of forceps, which is generally not difficult, removal of tartar from sound neighbouring teeth, and the adoption of measures already indicated for cleansing and purifying the mouth. Bleeding from the gum after extraction is of no importance and may safely be trusted to cease spontaneously. After removal of a carious tooth we must strictly regulate the diet, firstly giving soft food such as will require little mastication, and afterwards adopting a rational course of diet so as to give the teeth a fair amount of work and prevent others from becoming carious. To very nervous patients when suffering from toothache small doses of chlorodyne may be given; but it must be also remembered that fresh air and regular diet are the best means of correcting the neuralgiæ to which our pampered canine patients are so liable.

ABSCESS OF THE JAW is one of the most serious consequences of neglected caries of the fang. On removal of the tooth pus escapes and the healing process proceeds with rapidity, but sometimes this condition is neglected and severe osteitis sets in, a great deal of swelling of the bone is found; this is spongy, and the animal evidently suffers very much pain; there is profuse salivation, and entire refusal of food. At a later stage the abscess may burst below the jaw, leaving a fistulous ulcer running from below upwards. The gums become spongy, swollen, and very liable to bleed on the slightest touch, and the mouth is very offensive. This diseased state of the jaw is known as CANKER OF THE MOUTH, but as there is no specific influence at work this is not a good name for the affection. Of course sarcomatous disease may involve the jaw as well as any other bone in the body, and the irritation from a carious tooth may act as a determining cause, but the nonspecific disease is that which is seen in nine cases out of ten. *Treatment.*—Remove all carious teeth and evacuate any pus which has accumulated. Wash the mouth out regularly with solution of chloride of zinc. Dress the abscess cavity with tincture of myrrh. In the meanwhile strengthen the patient with tonics and easily digestible food, for this disorder is most exhausting.

No such serious effects from overgrowth follow the *loss of molar teeth* in the dog as in herbivora, the alveolus closes and becomes covered with a somewhat hardened gum, which, if not useful, is at any rate neutral in mastication.

CLEFT PALATE.—A curious case of this defect in development has come under my notice. The patient was a young bull terrier, and the central upper incisors were shed. The cloven condition of the palate was associated with harelip and a complete division between the two anterior nares. The defect apparently caused little inconvenience except the loss of incisor teeth due to atrophy of their fangs.

DISEASES OF THE TONGUE.—GLOSSITIS originates from injuries, such as stings, lacerations by sharp things seized by animals when enraged, burns, and bruising between the teeth. There is swelling of the organ, which hangs from the mouth in a state of temporary paralysis; some soreness of the throat is generally present, and saliva flows profusely from the mouth. Fever often runs high. *Treatment.*—Usually the acute symptoms rapidly subside if the patient be kept quiet, allowed a quantity of nitrated water to moisten his mouth with when he wishes, and not troubled by frequent administration of medicines or forcing with food. The functional importance of the affected organ is mainly in the direction of ingestion of water, and it is seldom inflamed except as a result of injury. Inflammation therefore subsides as the healing process of the wounded parts sets in, and chronic disorder of the organ seldom occurs.

In some animals PARALYSIS OF THE TONGUE, as indicated by its hanging constantly out of the mouth at one side in a dry, discoloured state, is seen. It no longer projects in a moist, healthy state, vibrating freely at its tip and edges, and ever and anon passing over the nose to renew its moisture. The animal suffers much from thirst (although lapping is not much interfered with) and experiences considerable discomfort. Breed seems to predispose to this disorder, animals of the bull-dog breed and spaniels having been found most liable to it. The paralysis is almost always unilateral and may generally be traced to injury or nervous disorder. It is to be treated by strict attention to hygiene and free administration of tonics, especially those, such as strychnia, which act particularly on the nervous system. This condition is sometimes congenital; it is generally incurable. It should be carefully guarded against in purchase of a valuable dog, for low-class fanciers in such cases remove the unsightliness by clipping off the protruding portion.

Wounds of the tongue must be treated on strictly conservative principles. It is said that the Greenlanders get rid of wolves by smearing sharp blades with blood which is frozen at once. The wolves in the act of licking it off lose the sensation in their tongues, which become seriously cut and useless; the wolf wastes away, and is ultimately eaten by its fellows. *Punctured wounds* through the tongue are sometimes caused by the tushes, and this organ may be seriously mangled in the course of an epileptic attack; but fortunately its wounds heal very readily.

Under the name of BLAIN, Youatt describes a vesicular affection of the lateral and under part of the tongue, which he tells us is seen also in the horse and ox, assuming a very great severity in the latter animal. In the dog it is often unaccompanied by other disease, there being simply a very profuse salivary flow, which ultimately becomes bloody and fetid, the tongue being raised from its base by intermaxillary swelling. He surmises that it originates as obstruction of the ducts of the sublingual salivary (!) glands (he evidently was not aware that there are none in the dog), and suggests free incisions into the vesicles and frequent washing of the mouth with a diluted solution of chlorinated lime, one part of the saturated solution and eleven of water, and subsequent astringent lotions. Generally tonics and nourishing food are required. Youatt says the disease is most frequent in spring and summer, and usually assumes an epidemic form. It is evident that, at any rate as concerns cattle, he wrote about foot-and-mouth disease. I have not seen any cases of this disorder; Hill mentions it, but his account reads like a copy of Youatt.

RANULA is sometimes seen in carnivores; in them the submaxillary gland is very large and the opening of its duct is apt to become occluded, whether by congestion of the mucous membrane in the mouth or by concretions. Then a globular swelling like a cyst appears beneath the front of the tongue. It may be removed by incision and is not likely to recur. The salivary apparatus is well developed and active in the dog as compared with the amount of starchy elements in his food, but the predominance in amount of saliva is of the viscid kinds of that fluid which perform mechanical functions, such as to keep the mouth moist and to lubricate the food passages.

PTYALISM, or *hypersalivation*, is the result of too free use of mercury compounds, whether internally or externally; in the latter case especially when the raw condition of the skin in an advanced stage of mange has not been fully considered. The mercury causes soreness of the gums, looseness and discolouration of the teeth, swelling of the salivary glands, fetor of the saliva, and disease of the bones, which will hereafter be considered. It also may give rise to such constitutional symptoms as will be mentioned under the heading "Mercurial Poisoning." It must be remembered that profuse salivation is often due to disease of the mouth. The history of the case must lead us to a correct diagnosis. In cases of ptyalism due to mercury poisoning small doses of iodide of potassium prove markedly beneficial. The free administration of dilute sulphuric acid is also advocated.

ULCERATION OF THE LIPS of a phagedænic character is not infrequent; there is much loss of substance, which is replaced by a flocculent mucoid substance. This is generally attributed to local injury and abrasions from tartar; but I am by no means convinced that this is the true cause, as even after apparent cure these ulcers are liable to recur and the parts involved remain hardened. They somewhat remind me of the ulcers on the lips of horses as seen during the "rains" in India, and of those of stomatitis gangrenosa as seen in the calf. *Treatment* consists in tonic doses and strict hygiene, cleansing of the mouth, and application of nitrate of silver to the ulcers; if there be marked indigestion the bowels must first be opened freely.

WARTS IN THE MOUTH invading the cheek, tongue, palate, and lips sometimes prove very troublesome for they are liable to become large and to disfigure the animal. They are generally so numerous as to defy thorough and complete removal with scissors, but this must be done as much as possible, and the operation repeated as often as necessary. The mouth also should be constantly rinsed out with a solution of acetic acid (1 to 40).

PHARYNGITIS has already been described in some detail under the heading "Sore-throat." We may supplement the remarks there made by saying that the pharynx is seldom the sole seat of inflammation. The disease may assume a chronic character, the parts becoming relaxed and swallowing requiring an effort for its proper accomplishment. In such cases there may be also thickening or ulceration of the lining membrane of the pharynx, and nitrate of silver must be applied as extensively as possible, the mouth being kept open with a gag and a long caustic holder used.

The œsophagus of the dog is large in calibre and highly dilatable, funnel-shaped at its posterior extremity, and red to its termination; there is free communication forwards as well as backwards between the stomach and the gullet. The stomach is relatively large, its lining mucous membrane is villous throughout, it has no well-marked blind pouch at the left extremity. The bowels are about five times the length of the body, one fifth being "large." They are simple (have no muscular bands or sacculi), the large and small differ little in size; the glands are well developed, the cæcum resembles the finger of a glove and is somewhat spirally twisted on itself, more so in some cases than in others. The wall of the rectum presents on each side a sinus of Morgagni, a glandular pouch from which a dark-coloured fetid matter is poured. The bowels of the dog are, therefore, short, straight, uniform in calibre throughout, simple as regards their shape, but composed of well-developed, highly organised structures.

Diseases and accidents of the Œsophagus: STRICTURE is sometimes seen as a result of injury to the lining membrane by bones or other hard bodies passing to the stomach, also after severe cases of choking, and as a result of the ravages of parasites (*Filaria sanguinolenta*). It is denoted by frequent slight attacks of choking, relieved spontaneously. Its ill effects may be palliated by soft, well-prepared food only being given. It is a serious matter in sporting dogs and others which require high feeding.

CHOKING.—The large size of the œsophagus enables masses of flesh, skin, and other such matters to pass freely into the stomach because the dog naturally bolts his food. Thus obstruction and mischief from foreign bodies is very often seen in the orifices of the stomach and in the bowels. Sometimes, however, sharp articles or those of an irregular shape become stopped in their passage through the gullet and give rise to choking. The pharyngeal orifice is sometimes the seat of impediment. The *symptoms* are not so urgent as in most other animals; there is obstruction to the passage of food, frequent attempts to regurgitate (which might be mistaken for vomiting), evident discomfort of the animal, cough, free flow of saliva, and perhaps some external swelling. Anything which is large enough to cause obstruction by its bulk will produce swelling visible to the eye, but small sharp objects become fixed by penetration of the walls of the œsophagus. In choking of the dog we therefore generally have some

ON THE DISORDERS OF THE DIGESTIVE APPARATUS. 109

degree of laceration to combat as well as the actual impaction; also the obstruction to the passage is generally only partial. In spite of the highly nervous temperament

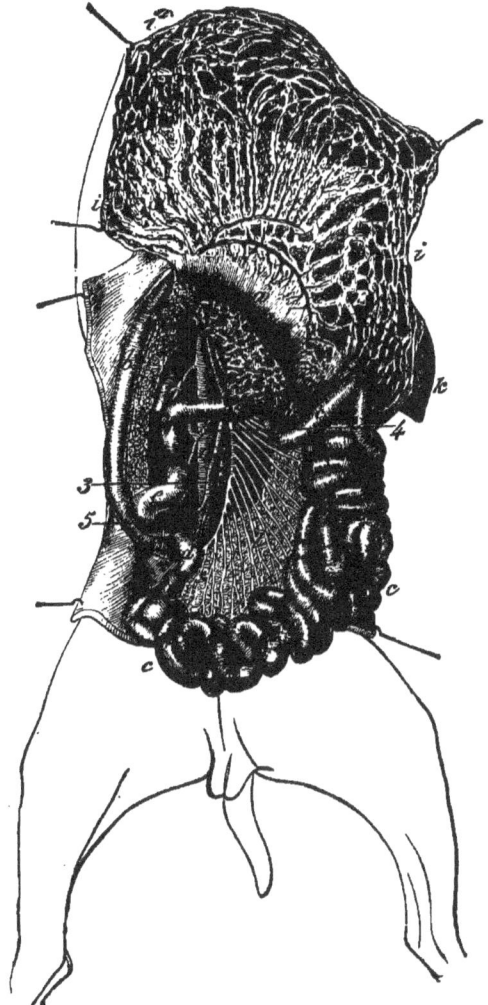

FIG. 34.—Intestines and omentum major (after CHAUVEAU).

a. Stomach. b. Duodenum. c, d. Small intestine. e. Cæcum. f, g, h. Large intestine. i. Omentum. k. Liver. l. Mesentery. m. Pancreas. 1. Post. aorta. 3, 4, 5. Intestinal branches of artery.

of some of our patients we do not often have to deal with œsophageal spasm. Bearing in mind these facts, we must not resort to extensive manipulation in these cases. An attempt may be made with Arnold's choking forceps (*vide*

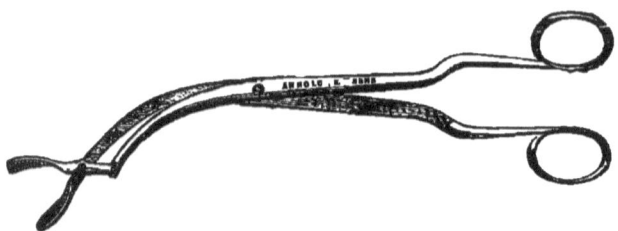

FIG. 35.—Throat forceps.

Fig. 35) to remove the foreign body, which will more readily pass upwards than down.* If this does not prove successful a large whalebone probe, used as a probang, may be passed into the œsophagus, and gentle pressure applied with a view to loosening the body from its position, but not with such energy as to lacerate still further the lining mucous membrane. The probe may be sheathed with a pad of tow dipped in oil for lubrication of the passage. *Œsophagotomy*, however, may be freely resorted to in these cases. Experience shows that wounds of the gullet of carnivora heal freely, probably because that organ is seldom put to its utmost degree of tension in the passage of prepared food; also, be it remembered, that probably in these cases one of the œsophageal coats is already cut through. The operation differs in no respect from the ordinary method, and it seems that sutures of the œsophageal wound are superfluous; after-treatment comprises attention to the external wound and fluid diet for a time.†

* Mr. Ward has recorded a case in a bull bitch which simulated dumb madness. There was some submaxillary swelling, and pressure on the base of the tongue with forceps caused escape of pus and blood, but from whence it was not possible to say. In a week's time a needle and cotton came away through the submaxillary abscess.

† It is to be remarked that fish-bones, needles, and other sharp hard substances not unfrequently pass through the walls of the œsophagus and the

ON SOME GENERAL SYMPTOMS OF DISORDER OF THE ALIMENTARY CANAL.—There are some conditions which, although generally described as disease, must be rather treated of as groups of symptoms which are usually due to derangement of the alimentary canal and its appendages, but may depend on disorder of other parts of the body or of the constitution in general. INAPPETANCE may be due to disinclination for food. It is often seen in pampered animals as a result of overfeeding or daintiness, or because the food offered is not tempting to the palate. It is one of the most frequent general indications of disorder, or it may depend on impediment such as choking, sore mouth, diseased teeth, or paralysis of the muscles of the jaws. The *treatment* consists in discovering and removing the cause.

INDIGESTION is very common in dogs : in the uncared for as a result of coarse indigestible food, in the over-cared for from too much and improper food, want of exercise, and general inattention to hygienic conditions. It is sometimes an indication of worms or foreign bodies in the stomach ; in other cases may depend on torpidity of the liver. It is an almost invariable accompaniment of advanced stages of debilitating disorders. Derangement of the teeth may be the cause, and it is almost always found that in these cases there are accumulations of tartar, softness of the gums, very foul breath, and dry, discoloured condition of the tongue. The appetite is depraved, the animal eats grass freely and vomits often, colicky pains, persistent constipation, and flatulence cause the animal serious inconvenience ; he is peevish, dull, and evidently out of sorts, and his coat feels harsh. In chronic cases the hair falls off and asthmatic symptoms set in ; sometimes animals which suffer from chronic indigestion are very fat. We need not here specify the *details of treatment*, for they comprise a removal, by medicine or otherwise, of the disorder on which the indigestion depends, and where this is not dis-

skin covering it. MacGillivray, of Banff, reminds us that the absence of sub-scapulo-hyoidean muscle from the dog facilitates cutting down on the œsophagus (' Vet. Journ.,' Jan., 1878).

tinctly recognisable we must content ourselves with strict attention to hygiene, tonics, and occasional laxatives. The alkaline carbonates are very useful in these cases, especially when the stomach is disordered, for in the dog there is a tendency to acidity and to the condition termed *pyrosis*, in which the stomach is irritable, and there is frequent ejection of a quantity of acid liquid through the mouth.

VOMITION.—The spasmodic ejection of the contents of the stomach depends either on the food being irritant, the stomach irritable, or the nervous system deranged. It is a symptom which may appear in almost any disease to which the dog is liable, so extensive are the reflex influences by which disorders of other parts derange the stomach. Because this process can be brought about in the dog by very many medicines, and the effect of emetics is one appreciable even to the most ignorant observer, this class of remedies has been much abused by those who have the care of sick dogs, emetics being given for every disease. They exhaust the patient and so indirectly exert a sedative influence, and they sometimes free the stomach of an irritant which is causing disease, but their use in canine medicine requires care and judgment.

PERSISTENT VOMITION is generally indicative of gastric disorder, but in fits of all kinds one of the earliest symptoms is a clearance of the stomach in this way. The matter ejected varies in different cases, the ordinary stomach contents being sometimes mixed with blood or a large quantity of bile. The inverse peristalsis occasionally extends to the bowels, and the pylorus becomes relaxed, which will account for the presence of bile in the vomits. The dog often eats grass as an emetic when he feels "sickness of the stomach." A very extreme case of vomition is recorded in the 'Abstract of Proceedings of the Veterinary Medical Association London, for 1838-9,' where the stomach was intussuscepted into the posterior end of the œsophagus; the whole of the gullet was much enlarged. In cases of persistant vomition small doses of prussic acid or morphia and alkaline effervescent drinks must be tried.

Colic is the term applied to those symptoms which indicate that an animal is suffering from pain referable to the abdomen unassociated with inflammation. In true simple colic there is actually spasm of the bowels, such as may result from an irritant in the intestinal passage or even (through transference of reflex impressions) in some other part of the body, such as stomach or uterus. In other cases colicky symptoms depend on the presence of obstruction of the bowels as by calculus, impaction, or stricture, or disease of stomach, liver, bladder, or other abdominal organs. It may depend upon poisonous matters in the blood; thus one of the most prominent symptoms of lead poisoning is colic, and it often supervenes during the progress of an attack of distemper. Colic very frequently occurs in puppies, probably from alterations in quality of the mother's milk, and it is often seen in pregnant bitches, when it is the condition known as false labour-pains or else depends on pressure of the distended female generative organs on the neck of the bladder. Of all the irritants which may give rise to simple colic the most frequent are worms, indigestible matters, and sharp bones. *Symptoms.*—In some cases the invasion is very sudden, the animal exhibiting very marked signs of pain, but usually the first manifestations are those of a sense of discomfort, the animal moans in its sleep, awakes suddenly, lies down, curls himself up, and goes to sleep again. This continues until at last the paroxysms are too urgent to allow of repose while they last. The patient utters sharp, shrill, continuous cries; tries all sorts of positions to give himself ease, and walks about with his back arched. There may be a distended state of the abdomen due to flatulence. Blaine speaks of a form of colic which occurs in cases of rheumatism. *Treatment.*—Having assured ourselves that no fever is present, and examined the condition of the fæces, if any, and explored the abdominal contents by firm pressure and manipulation of the belly to ascertain whether any tumour or accumulation is the cause of colic, it is as well to at once resort to a warm bath and active friction of the surface. This often affords much relief; it may be followed by an emetic to remove possible causes of irritation from the stomach, and soap-and-water enemata at intervals of an hour. If the pain is very urgent an anodyne antispasmodic draught should be given and repeated every two hours as long as necessary. In almost every case an oleaginous cathartic is indicated. When the pain is severe and the paroxysms prove frequent and of long duration, mustard plasters or stimulating liniment may be applied to the belly; but in all these cases of colic we must carefully ascertain on what disorder the abdominal pain depends, and must direct our efforts to removal of that disorder. About forty minims of laudanum with a dessertspoonful of strong brandy and water, is a good colic drink for routine practice. The flatulent form of colic is very rare in carnivora.

DIARRHŒA.—The frequent passage of fluid fæces exceeding the normal in total bulk, differs from "looseness of the bowels," in which the fæces are simply abnormally soft. In cases of diarrhœa, tenesmus and colic are generally present; in chronic diarrhœa, indigestion, debility, and often ulceration of the bowel against the anus, with relaxation of the sphincter, are present. Acute cases may be catarrh of the bowels induced by the presence of some irritant leading to increased secretion from the various highly developed intestinal glands, and also from the mucous membrane. This irritant may be food, worms, acrid bile, &c., or the catarrh may be due to changes in the weather, or to disorder of the blood. Diarrhœa also may be simply a culmination of debilitating disease and carry off the patient, or it may depend on hyper-secretion of bile, or on abuse of purgative medicine (when it is termed "super-purgation"). *Treatment.*—These cases always require careful nursing, and when they become chronic are apt to assume a dysenteric character. Cleanliness, the giving of food of a readily digestible nature, and avoidance of exposure, are particularly to be attended to. Often an aperient is in the commencement necessary for removal of acrid matters from the alimentary canal;

oleaginous cathartics, as sheathing the membrane, are specially indicated. In chronic or persistent cases the animal must be given astringent diet and doses of tonics carefully regulated and given with astringents and antacids. Glycerine, vaseline, or oleaginous applications round the anus, will save the animal much pain. In cases where there is extensive intestinal disease, but little can be done although tonics afford the best chance of temporary relief from exhausting diarrhœa. Diarrhœa proves very fatal to puppies, and in them it requires very careful treatment. The bitch must be kept quiet and her diet regulated lest aperient principles affect the pups through the milk. A frequent examination of the character of the stools will prove our best guide in determining the exact seat of the mischief in these cases; if the liver be acting more freely than usual, the fæces will be very dark coloured and offensive, in such cases, as well as when a deficiency of colouring matter in the dung indicates torpidity, calomel or podophyllin in small doses will prove useful.

CONSTIPATION, COSTIVENESS, AND TORPIDITY OF THE BOWELS are conditions varying in degree rather than in kind; an animal being constipated when he passes no fæces; costive when he passes hard fæces with much effort, and in torpidity of the bowels the peristalsis is retarded and the bowels act infrequently, the fæces being unusually dry from retention. The natural stimuli to intestinal movements are diet, a free supply of bile, and exercise. If the food be given irregularly and contain a deficiency of vegetable matters costiveness will result. Among all carnivora there is an infrequency of action of the bowels and the fæces as passed are dry and hard, but some individuals are habitually costive and suffer much inconvenience; yard dogs and pets which are not allowed to walk sufficiently for exercise suffer from severe intestinal derangements as sequelæ of constipation. It must be remembered also that torpidity of the bowels is one of the most marked symptoms of the feverish state and of serious disorder of the alimentary canal or its appendages, especially the liver; a blunted nervous sense, so to speak, in some outdoor breeds seem to predispose to this irregularity. Costiveness pure and simple must be dealt with by a careful regulation of the diet into which some such laxative element as vegetables (cabbage especially) should occasionally enter; also liver, boiled or uncooked, may be given once a week; regular exercise and regular feeding must be enforced. Where the retention has become associated with extreme dryness of a large mass of fæces collected in the rectum, this may be detected by manipulation of the belly, the presence of abdominal pain, constant attempts to pass fæces only resulting in a bulging of the anal structures but with no relaxation of the sphincter. "The agony caused by costiveness is greater than in any other affection to which the dog is liable. Apparently well, and perhaps at play, a cry breaks forth which is the next instant a shriek, expressive of the acutest torture. The animal takes to running and is not aware of surrounding objects; it can recognise nothing, but will bite its master if he attempts to catch it, and hit itself against anything that may be in its way; it scampers from room to room, or hurries from place to place; it is unable to be still or silent, and perhaps getting into a corner it makes continuous efforts as though it wished to scramble up the wall, remaining there jumping with all its strength, and at the same time yelling at the top of its voice. This excitement may last for an hour or more, and then cease only to be renewed, till at length the powers fail, and in half a day the animal may be dead. Just prior to death a mass of compact fæces is usually passed, and blood, with dysentery, is generally witnessed for the short period the animal survives" (Mayhew). In such cases removal of the accumulated fæces with the oiled forefinger inserted *per anum* is indicated; the handle of a teaspoon will prove useful for breaking down the hardened mass, and small doses of oil and oleaginous or alkaline injections will materially assist. The bowels afterwards will require constant attention and careful regulation as this condition is liable to continually recur.

DISEASES OF THE STOMACH: GASTRIC CATARRH.

—The stomach of the dog, as being relatively of more importance as a digestive organ than that of the horse, is more liable to disorder. Its mucous lining membrane is extensive and highly organised, and consequently very liable to derangement. Dogs are often fed so erroneously, without regularity, indiscriminately on all sorts of diet, too often and with too much at a time, that we cannot wonder at gastric derangements being common. Parasites and foreign bodies of different kinds are frequent in the stomach, and constitute another source of disease. We have elsewhere noticed the condition of the stomach known as pyrosis, in which there is indigestion with profuse secretion from the gastric glands. We have now to examine a more definite disorder consisting in either congestion or inflammation of the lining mucous membrane. Some fever of a subacute character is present; there are all the phenomena of indigestion; the stomach is irritable and rejects promptly both food and medicine, also every now and then its contents are thrown up in the form of acid secretion without any admixture of food; there is pain on pressure over the seat of the stomach in the majority of these cases. Sooner or later the inflammation extends to the lining membrane of the bowels and diarrhœa sets in, and experience has shown that this is a very serious matter and very liable to lead to a fatal termination. Because there is cough present in most of these cases it has been termed *Husk*, but this name is objectionable since it has been for a long time applied to parasitic bronchitis of calves, and so some confusion might arise from the designation of an altogether distinct pathological state by a name having already a widespread popular use in reference to a particular disease. *Treatment* presents serious difficulties, the most important being that of retention of food or medicine, both of which must be bland and of small bulk, and therefore frequently administered. Dilute hydrocyanic acid (gtt. j to iij), chlorodyne, opium, are very valuable here, and the alkaline carbonates counteract the excessive acidity of the gastric secretion.

It must be our aim to gradually increase the tone and lessen the irritability of the stomach, and to this end liquid food containing sedative medicines must be given, and supplemented by nutrient enemata. In the chronic form of this disorder small doses of nux vomica may prove beneficial, but our main reliance must be on the vegetable tonics.

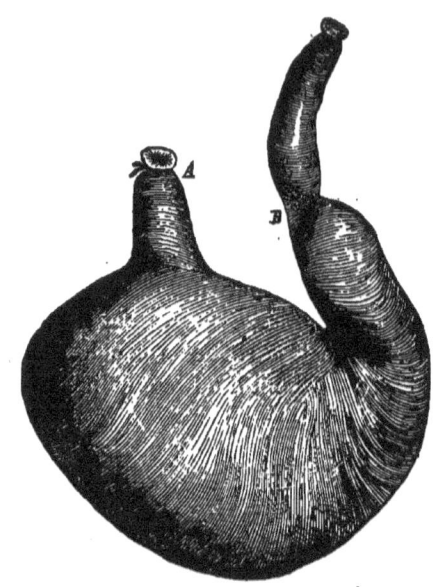

Fig. 36.—Stomach (After Chauveau).
A. Cardia, with œsophagus.   B. Pylorus, with duodenum.

Gastritis is that form of inflammation of the stomach which affects especially its muscular and mucous coats. It is seldom seen except as a result of irritant poisoning, although it has been in some cases attributed to external violence, the action of foreign bodies and exposure to inclement weather, &c. No doubt the stomach of the dog is much predisposed to disorder on account of the excessive demands made upon its digestive powers in artificial life; the wild dog is but slightly a vegetable feeder, whereas the tame dog is in many cases almost herbivorous, always omnivorous. The stomach has thus to digest matters for which it is not naturally adapted, but to which it has become habituated. But this perversion of function predisposes to disease, generally, however, of the lining membrane only. *Symptoms* develope gradually as those of indigestion, such as depraved appetite, a tendency to lick cool things, thirst, and frequent vomition. Fever subsequently sets in and the sickness is persistent. The animal tries to find a cool place to lie down on, pants severely, moans or whines frequently, and stretches himself out so that he can lie with his belly against the ground. There is pain on pressure over the stomach, and heat is distinctly perceptible. The tongue is especially dirty and foul in this disorder, and occasionally there is vomiting of blood (hæmatemesis). *Treatment.—* Good nursing is urgently required, frequent draughts of cool mucilaginous drinks with small doses of alkalies and sedatives. Poultices and free fomentation, or mustard plasters to the belly, and a free access to cold water for drinking. We shall hereafter mention some of the more frequent poisons and the manner in which their special effects may be counteracted. After resolution has set in, a course of alkalies and tonics will prove beneficial, and the greatest care must be exercised with a view to giving the animal's food only in small quantities at a time, and in a readily digestible form.

ULCER IN THE STOMACH is occasionally seen as an indication of malnutrition, and thus it may be a sequela of distemper or may depend on starvation and imprisonment in a dark, damp, unhealthy place. I have several times observed it under the latter conditions, and it is sometimes associated with ulceration of the cornea, identical in nature and causes.

GASTRIC FISTULA.—It is rather a favourite operation with physiologists to artificially induce a direct communication between the stomach cavity and the surface. It can be done in most cases with impunity, and valuable conclusions as to the physiology of gastric digestion have thus been arrived at. The patient lives and enjoys himself with the trochar extending through the abdominal and gastric walls. Gamgee describes the operation in detail.

GASTRIC DILATATION is often found post-mortem in old dogs which have become dyspeptic from a long course of over-feeding. The animal is liable to tympany and colic during life.

FOREIGN BODIES IN THE STOMACH* are either introduced through the œsophagus in their formed state, or gradually produced by mechanical and chemical forces from the materials ingested from without. When sharp and indigestible, foreign substances cause gastric fistula, and thus either escape through the walls of the belly or into the abdominal cavity among the bowels, where they may cause mischief: needles, forks, nails, &c., soon act in this way, and when they emerge from the fistula, or are extracted by operation, they are found to be more or less eroded by the action of the gastric juice. Rounded bodies of even considerable size can escape from the stomach into the bowels, the pylorus being somewhat lax towards the end of the process of gastric digestion, when it admits of a rush of such matters as the stomach has been unable to deal with. I consider that this can be physiologically accounted for, on the theory that masses of vegetable matter are not freely acted on in the stomach where there is a deficiency of glycogenic saliva, but must pass on to the bowels where it is subjected to the pancreatic secretion. Perhaps, however, there is a reflux of both pancreatic and biliary matters normally into the stomach of the dog to a limited extent. At any rate, it is wonderful what large foreign bodies, stones, jagged bones, and the like will pass from the stomach into the bowels in some cases. Animals taught to fetch and carry stones are apt to swallow them, puppies in their play, and probably as a result of teeth irritation, will swallow stones and dirt; pregnant bitches and animals with indigestion from other

* Raddell relates a case of a pointer which ate a small King Charles' spaniel and died from *ruptured stomach*. This is very curious on account of the rarity of the lesion and the cannibal tendencies of the subject. 'Veterinary Record,' iii, p. 129.

causes will eat dung, dirt, &c., and we are well aware that eating straws, pebbles, and the like, is one of the most marked signs of rabies. Again, small animals covered with hair may be eaten, cured skins may be gnawed, or even (as in a case recorded by Mr. Hill in the 'Veterinary Journal,' vol. x, p. 79) human hair combings may be ingested. These are felted by the peristaltic action of the stomach and glued together by mucus, and thus "hair-balls" are formed.* Indigestion, pure and simple, is generally the result of rounded concretions; if they be small they are expelled by vomition or passed onwards into the bowels, but if they be large they will give rise to chronic indigestion; saline-calcareous aggregations, true gastric calculi, are very rare in the dog. I will here mention observations by Mr. Hunting as made at the Central Veterinary Society at its Meeting on June 8th, 1882; he exhibited a small stone and a cork which he had taken from the stomachs of two dogs. The first was a small black and tan bitch, which was suddenly seized with vomiting and convulsions. Fits always followed the administration of solid food. The stomach having been diagnosed as the seat of mischief the patient was given Brand's essence of beef, as the only nutriment allowed, and, medicinally, hydrocyanic acid and bismuth trinitrate; some improvement occurred, but the animal was unable to take even beef-tea with a sediment without vomiting and died in a few days. The cork was

* Vol. iii of the 'Veterinary Journal' contains a record of the case of a valuable Esquimaux dog which was observed to be very dull, to hide in corners, and lie on his belly with his hind legs apart; pulse 150 and thready; vomition; nose hot and dry. On the evening of the following day symptoms of brain derangement set in, there was stiffness of gait, occasionally ineffectual attempts at vomition were made, and a severe convulsive fit occurred as night set in. On the third day the bowels had not acted, urine passed involuntarily, and some tetanic symptoms were present. Towards evening he crawled about on the belly, or hung back at the full length of his chain. He died at 12 midnight, in a very strong convulsive fit. Autopsy showed a cobble-stone, weighing about one ounce avoirdupois, lodged at the pyloric end of the greater curvature, causing inflammation and engorgement of the mucous membrane. Two pieces of white fibrous material, with a little flesh attached at one end, and a bit of yellowish fat at the other (chordæ tendinæ probably) were found loose in the right ventricle.

found firmly plugging the pyloric orifice, and the adjacent mucous membrane was much thickened and inflamed* * * * * The second dog had suffered more or less for six months, it became very thin and occasionally showed much distress, heaving at the flanks, and suffering from vomiting, fits, and convulsions. The stone found in the stomach was too large to pass into the intestines, and the pyloric orifice was rendered small by an excessive thickening of the coats of the stomach. Mr. Hunting draws attention to two clinical memoranda for such cases:—(1) The beef-tea made from Brand's essence being perfectly fluid, is the only form of nourishment which is retained in these instances. (2) It is only when the foreign body attempts to pass the pylorus that convulsions occur, or that irritation of the stomach which induces them.

Youatt ('The Dog,' 1861) quotes two remarkable cases in each of which a large dog swallowed a fork, and it could be felt by manipulation in the stomach. In the first case the veterinary surgeon judiciously kept the dog's stomach well distended by feeding him on cow's-liver and gave doses of dilute sulphuric acid. In due course a fistula formed and by the aid of incision the fork was removed, much corroded, and minus its ivory handle, which had been digested, and the animal did very well. In the second case, on abdominal incision the handle of the fork was found among the viscera, and the remainder embedded in the root of the mesocolon where it was causing much inflammatory mischief. This animal also recovered.

PARASITES IN THE STOMACH.—The most frequent worm seen in the stomach of the dog is *Ascaris marginata*, which is probably identical with *A. mystax* of the cat (Cobbold). They gain the stomach probably by migrating from the intestines and give rise to some irritation, and thus they become expelled by vomition, but they sometimes produce serious and even fatal effects. Thus in the 'Veterinarian,' 1878, p. 353, are mentioned two cases, in one of which five of these worms caused intussusception and rupture of the bowel in a puppy; in the other death resulted from their puncturing the duodenum. It is always well in cases of indigestion to give vermifuges suitable for both round-worms and tape-worms, as these are a frequent source of disorder, indeed, they may be the cause of epileptic fits in puppies. Oil of turpentine, common salt, santonin, or sulphate of iron are useful in such cases. *Spiroptera* (v. *Filaria*) *sanguinolenta* sometimes is seen in cystic abodes in the wall of the stomach of the dog. In the lining membrane of the stomach of the cat resides the adult *Olulanus tricuspis*, a trichina-like animal, the embryos of which either penetrate the liver and lungs, " the infested animal perishing in consequence of the inflammatory action set up by their presence," in some cases, or are passed with the fæces, and in the mouse develop just as trichina do in man.

We may here with advantage discuss the question *whether dogs should be allowed to feed on bones*, which frequently arises in the course of canine practice. It cannot be doubted that the ingestion of bones has a physiological value in all carnivora, they are taken freely by the animal and swallowed. They serve to clear the teeth from tartar accumulations, and possibly assist in gastric repletion and mild stimulation of the lining mucous membrane of the stomach, just as stones in a bird's gizzard do. They are digested freely and afford useful nutriment in the form of phosphates and bone gelatine. On the other hand they are a fruitful source of mischief, *firstly*, in breaking and displacing the teeth; *secondly*, in becoming impacted in the œsophagus and so choking the animal; *thirdly*, when sharp and spicular, in penetrating the wall of the œsophagus or stomach and so reaching the surface; *fourthly*, in causing impaction of the bowels, especially the large one. But, be it observed, it is not the size of the bone but its roughness and sharpness which causes this mischief; and so these ill-effects can not be attributed simply to the ingestion of them as bones but as sharp bodies liable to wound. We may conclude that the dog in health benefits considerably from an occasional feed of bones; he enjoys it, and it tends to improve his digestion; but these bones are to be given unbroken, and sharp fish bones are liable to cause trouble with toy dogs; the occasional feed of bones ought to be *de rigueur*.

DISEASES OF THE INTESTINES: ENTERITIS.—True inflammation of the bowels is more frequent in the dog than in the horse; although by some authorities it is said to be "very common," this cannot be considered correct, but the result of opinion based on imperfect diagnosis; essentially there is a certain amount of gastritis in these cases. The muscular coat of the bowel is the main seat of disorder, and this accounts for obstinate torpidity of the bowels being a very marked symptom. The most frequent causes of enteritis are impaction, intussusception, or some form of strangulation of the bowels. Next in importance to these rank irritant poisonous substances, and it is said that exposure to cold, as from lying through the night on a bed of wet straw or on damp earth, exposure to a cutting wind when the coat has recently been removed, overexertion, and other such deleterious influences act as causes. Mayhew has noticed that it is very frequent as a result of maltreatment of cases of mange by excessively powerful stimulants.

Symptoms.—So urgent is the distress in these cases, and so altered the general behaviour of the animal, that they have been mistaken for rabies, especially as the eyes are very red, the voice is altered by pain, and paralysis sets in in the later stages of the attack. Fever commences with a shivering fit and then seems very high; there is obstinate and continuous abdominal pain, and the animal cries with agony when the belly is pressed upon, yet he may gently press this part against the ground in the hope to find ease. Generally, however, he runs away to some dark quiet place and lies flat on his side panting and crying. On manipulation the belly is found to be hot, and the animal is likely to snap when it is pressed upon. No fæces is passed and the urine is generally very scanty and high coloured. There is a hardness and smallness about the pulse, and the tail is carried pressed down over the anus. *Treatment* is seldom successful, for the inflammation runs on quickly to gangrene, as denoted by cessation of pain and the supervention of all the symptoms of collapse. It has been remarked by Mayhew that in this disease there is a special disinclination to take any medicines. Cases have been known in which intussusception was relieved by means of *laparotomy*, surgical incision into the abdomen and mechanical freeing of the bowel, and in other cases the entangled piece has sloughed off and resolution set in; but such cases are rare. Our first care must be to determine by the history of the case or else by digital exploration through the fundament, the cause of inflammation. Enemata of warm water and soap must be freely given, or when there is a tendency to accumulation of hard fæces they must be broken down and removed in the manner already indicated, and an enema of some bland oil then given. No purgative must be resorted to when the disease has fully established itself, except a full dose of olive or other such oil, the tendency of which is to act mechanically by admixture with hard fæces, and so much of it as is digested and absorbed proves nutritive; also the stomach, though somewhat intolerant, will retain it. Crude opium, chlorodyne, or Indian hemp must be given internally to allay pain and to exert some sedative influence on the circulation. A warm bath has proved highly beneficial in such cases, and free fomentation, as also application of linseed poultices to the belly, is indicated. Blaine says : " Dogs are very liable to rheumatism, but it is no less true than curious that a dog never has acute, and seldom chronic rheumatism either, that is not accompanied, more or less, with inflammation of his bowels; this connection of diseases is, however, as far as my experience goes, confined to the dog alone. In many cases the bowels are the immediate and principal seat of the rheumatism, which is productive of a peculiar enteritis, easily distinguished by those conversant with the diseases of dogs." In this, as in numbers of other conclusions, Blaine's original observations have not been thoroughly accepted by subsequent observers.

DYSENTERY.—Is true inflammation of the mucous lining membrane of the bowels—the effect of prolonged use of innutritious food, of neglected diarrhœa, of the too continued use of irritant medicines, and, it is said, acridity of the bile also causes it. *Symptoms.*—Diarrhœa, the ejecta being of an extremely offensive character often tinged with blood, containing very hard small lumps, and often much frothy or stringy mucus. They have an acridity which leads to excoriation around the anus and to frequent tenesmus. The animal suffers from fever and abdominal pain, and there is rapidly increasing emaciation, so that very soon after the commencement of the attack the patient is in an extreme state of debility, and its breath and cutaneous emanations smell foul and sickly. Sometimes a considerable amount of blood is passed with the stools. Where the dysentery is subacute, the result of chronicity of diarrhæa, the animal becomes a most miserable object, a living skeleton, generally covered with external parasites, and filthy about the anus. Occasionally the stomach is involved in this disorder by the continuity of its structure with that of the bowel, then persistent vomition is a marked symptom, although the appetite may be ravenous and depraved. Paralysis usually sets in several days before death.

Treatment of this serious disorder requires to be prolonged and very careful. Husbanding the strength by every available means is necessary. Broth, milk, cod-liver oil, and other nutritives may be given by the mouth and also, mixed with astringents, *per anum*. When the animal is in much pain opium (1—3 grs.) must be given every second hour until ease is obtained. I prefer for continued administration the astringent tonic barks, such as oak and cinchona, and with them may be combined a little chalk. The dilute mineral acids form tonic drinks which are useful and palatable in these cases. Astringent suppositories (medicines introduced by means of the finger *per anum*) are useful, and infusion of gentian, catechu, or oak galls may be given as enemata frequently. But our main reliance must be on cleanliness, fresh air, gentle exercise, and good generous diet; in fact, this is a disease in the treatment of which everything rests on good nursing.

We have next to deal with a number of surgical conditions, such as are rather frequent in the dog and generally very serious.

IMPACTION is denoted by colicky pains, which are somewhat more continuous than those of simple colic, and are followed by enteritis: external manipulation or digital rectal exploration may enable us to detect some obstructing mass. Generally obstinate constipation is present, and not unfrequently some vomiting. The offending substance varies in different cases, thus sometimes it is a bone, sometimes a stercoral mass, or an accumulation of vegetable matter, or a stone which has been swallowed. Occasionally, perhaps, a *calculus*; but this kind of impediment is very rare in the dog, for there are no sacculi of the walls of the bowels of carnivora in which such concretions can seclude themselves and oppose the propulsive movements of peristalsis.* In cases where we are sure impactment of some kind is present, and relief does not follow treatment with antispasmodics, *laparotomy* should be performed before the strength of the animal fails. Dogs are very tolerant of this operation. I have no evidence of *Volvulus* occurring in the dog—probably the shortness and directness of the bowels has something to do with this. But, on the other hand, INVAGINATION or INTUSSUSCEPTION is very frequent, probably because reversed peristalsis can occur as readily in the bowels as in the œsophagus of the dog. Large dogs seem most prone to this derangement, a fact which must be remembered in dealing with cases of intestinal obstruction in them. The most frequent form of invagination is where the cæcum, carrying with it the terminal portion of the ileum, passes into the cavity of the colon. It is really wonderful how little urgency is shown from the symptoms in these cases, and often after death there is no trace of adhesions about

* Youatt quotes a case in which a sacculus had formed in the wall of the ileum and accommodated the calculus.

the invaginated bowel. In other cases, however, we have the symptoms of enteritis complicated by those of bile resorption, and if the animal does not succumb, it is found that after the lapse of a considerable time the impacted piece of bowel is thrown off as a slough and expelled *per anum*. I think it must be accepted as an axiom in canine surgery that where intestinal obstruction is marked and obstinate, laparotomy should be performed before the powers of the patient flag. Cases have been known in which, with antiseptic precautions, a couple of inches of bowel have been freed from the rest by two incisions, and the cut ends of the bowel, thus shortened, having been brought together and retained by suture, have re-united, the excised portion being utilised by the experimenter for collection of succus entericus. Youatt tells us that enteritis will not long exist without leading to intussusception. Mayhew considers the cæcum the main seat of intestinal disease in most cases; he says: "In the dog which has died of intestinal disease, the cæcum is almost invariably found enlarged and inflamed. In it I imagine the majority of bowel affections have their origin. The gut is first loaded, and the consequence of this is it loses its natural function. The contents become irritants from being retained, and the whole process of digestion is deranged; other parts are involved and inflammation is induced."

PROLAPSUS RECTI *vel Ani* is a result of debility, and consists in protrusion of a portion of the rectum through the anal opening. Either all the coats of the bowel are extruded or only the mucous, which has become much relaxed. This "dropping of the bowel" is most frequently seen in old dogs, and is in the majority of instances a result of the costive habit. The protruded portion seldom becomes strangulated but gradually undergoes changes which increase the difficulty in replacing it and favour its reprotrusion. The bowel must be promptly returned after cleansing, and cold astringent applications and astringent suppositories or injections resorted to for several days. Also the animal should be fed on boiled rice and soup for some time after the accident. In chronic cases excision is necessary, and may be boldly resorted to, either by means of the hot iron or by the knife, and the use of the interrupted suture. Mayhew, however, prefers to excise a circular portion of the lining membrane only. To prevent this and other ill-effects of constipation animals of a costive habit should have periodically a feed of unboiled liver or of boiled greens, podophyllin pills may also be tried.

HÆMORRHOIDS or PILES are often seen in the dog, being associated with old age, habitual costiveness, and general laxity of the alimentary canal. They are found as tumours external to the bowel, or only protruded when the anus projects after evacuation of fæces; sometimes they render the margin of the anal opening unsightly and irregular. They are sero-sanguineous, or semi-solid, tumours generally highly vascular. Sooner or later they become sluggish, irritable ulcers. Treatment consists in removal by ligature, taking measures for prevention of costiveness, and, in the case of internal piles, astringent suppositories. It is to be remarked that bleeding piles are less frequent in the dog than in man, although occasionally seen; that the liver is less frequently a cause of piles in the dog than in man; and, finally, that piles should always be looked for very carefully in examination of dogs as to soundness. They are very liable to be aggravated and prematurely opened by the animal drawing the anus along the ground while walking along on his forelegs, as he is apt to do when the anus is irritable from any cause. *Fistula in Ano* is a result of neglected piles or laceration of the lining membrane of the rectum by sharp impacted bones, or its abrasion by means of very dry, hard fæces. It may need operative interference, but generally measures which tend to hasten evacuation of the rectum, and to keep its contents soft, are sufficient; thus oleaginous enemata are useful. Possibly the sinuses of Morgagni have at times been mistaken for fistulæ. The rectum is liable to *atony*, especially in old dogs which do not get much exercise. The fæces accumulate in the rectum and get very hard, there is a foul smelling discharge from the sebaceous glands of the anus, and the margin of the opening becomes dry, harsh, and ulcerated; œdema of the perinæum may occur as a result. This is seen in chronic diarrhœa and as a complication in cases of dysentery. It must be treated by means of tonic astringent enemata, and the administration through the mouth of tonics and laxatives; also occasional mechanical removal of hard masses of fæces from the rectum. Mayhew's remarks upon pathological states of the terminal portion of the bowel are excellent.

POLYPUS RECTI is a disease of not infrequent occurrence. The tumour is generally removeable by ligature, and probably the growths described under this name are merely large hard piles.

STRICTURE OF THE BOWEL is rather frequent, indeed Mr. A. Broad, a well-known London canine practitioner, considers "induration and thickening of the commencing portion of the duodenum very common in dogs," and there are numerous cases of stricture, with or without consequent dilatation, on record. Such may account for obscure intermittent colic; they mainly result from chemical or mechanical irritants causing a shrinking scar of the lining membrane of the bowel. They are seldom or never curable, but, if suspected, may be palliated by the routine adoption of a soft laxative diet.

HERNIA ABDOMINALIS.—The several forms of hernia of the intestines and their appendages as seen in man, are not very frequent in the dog, because of the simplicity of the bowels and their short length. *Epiplocele* in puppies is not infrequent, the protrusion taking place through the umbilical opening. The exploring needle having been used, the omentum may be cut down on and excised or else returned into the belly and retained by a truss or by a ligature round the neck of the hernial sac. However, it is a matter of difficulty to keep on a truss, and the method of excision is not liable to any serious complication, so I am inclined to prefer the latter. *Femoral and Inguinal Herniæ* are seen in bitches especially, the contents being bowels, horns of uterus, or bladder. Hill, in the 'Veterinary Journal,' vol. vii, p. 236, relates a most interesting successful case of operative interference in double inguinal hernia, the contents of one sac being the bowel, those of the other bowel and bladder. Vol. i, p. 62, of the same periodical contains an interesting case by Friederberger of similar character but fatal result of operative interference under chloroform. Death was attributed to commencing septicæmia, and disturbance of the circulation through the brain and lungs, due to too prompt return of the organs, both sides having been operated on simultaneously. I have to hand an interesting specimen of *Ventral Hernia* in which the uterus constitutes the protruding organ. These accidents almost always result from injury, and must be treated on ordinary surgical principles; prolapsus and invagination are, however, the forms of intestinal ectopia most frequently seen in the dog.

WORMS IN THE BOWELS.—The intestines are the frequent abode of animals of numerous species belonging to the genera Nematoda and Cestoda, commonly known as round- and tape-worms. It is natural to these worms to live there, but sometimes a source of much discomfort to the dog and animals associated with him. The discomfort to the animal himself is caused by the activity of the parasites in pursuit of their everyday occupations, seldom by the mechanical ill-effects of their presence. We have seen that the dog is as a rule of high nervous organisation; this renders him liable to reflex paralysis, cough, and convulsions from irritation caused by worms in the bowels. More often, however, the manifestations are those which follow mild stimulation of the lining membrane of the bowels persistent to a disordering degree. Depraved appetite and unthriftiness, a harsh unhealthy state of the skin, loss of hair, progressive anæmia, irregularity of the bowels, the fæces offensive, slimy, and infested with parasites. There is generally a certain amount of irritation of the anus, which renders the animal fond of licking that part or dragging it along the ground. Sometimes the worms migrate from the bowel into the stomach, and are expelled by vomition. In other cases persistent diarrhœa and obstinate indigestion may be traced to the presence of worms, or the growth of young animals may be checked in spite of the consumption of an extraordinary amount of food. The "worms" most frequently seen in the fæces of the dog are actively moving shortly after expulsion, and look like small round worms. They are known in kennels as "maw-worms," and are really mature segments of tapeworms full of eggs ready to be hatched. Those worms which are expelled by vomition are round, and the same (*Ascaris marginata*) as have already been mentioned under the heading "Worms in the Stomach." They sometimes migrate even farther, and cases have been known in which they have caused death by entering into the air-passages; such an occurrence is, of course, very rare. Because an animal which has died in convulsions or paralysed is found to have a worm in his bowels this is by no means the only possible cause of death, indeed we should examine most carefully for all other possible causes, remembering that the presence of even a number of worms in the bowels is quite compatible with robust health. Either these worms prefer to inhabit young animals, or, as they cause disease more often in young than in old, we are apt to consider them most liable to affect puppies; the latter is the most probable. We are by no means well informed about the life-history of round-worms, many of them probably require no intermediary bearer, and it is certain that they appear in animals which live with infested dogs. Even milk-drinking puppies shortly after birth have been found to have round-worms in their stomachs. From this we learn that such worms and the fæces of dogs having them ought to be burned. Santonin is the vermifuge best adapted for the removal of these worms, given in doses of three to five grains. Dr. Cobbold introduced it into canine practice; he insists that it should be given with a full dose of castor-oil and followed by the exhibition of tonics, and that salt and water, carbolic solutions, and bucketfuls of boiling water ought to be thrown over the floors of the kennels. Three other forms of round-worms are found in the intestines of the dog, but are of much less clinical importance than Ascaris :—

1. *Dochmius trigonocephalus*, found in the stomach and intestine.
2. *Tricocephalus depressiusculus*, found in the cæcum.
3. *Trichina spiralis* has been, experimentally, developed in the intestines (and muscles) of the dog.*

The tapeworms of the dog are numerous and important. It must be remembered that an animal is not free from them until the head, apparently the most insignificant part, has passed; so long as this remains attached to the wall of the bowel will it develop fresh egg-producing segments, which are passed *per vias naturales* and prove the means of diffusion of the parasite.

Great as are the inconveniences and other troubles produced by the mature tapeworms, their larvæ, known as cystic worms, are much more serious, especially from the point of view of comparative pathology. We may proceed to notice, *seriatim*, the tæniæ of the dog in so far as they have a practical bearing on pathology.

1. *T. cucumerina*, so called from its cucumber-shaped segments. It inhabits the small intestines, is a small but very long tapeworm, the segments of which separate when mature, escape through the anus, and then discharge their ova in the coat of the dog, which are ingested by the dog-louse, *Trichodectes latūs*.

2. *T. cænurus* is found in the small intestines. Its ova fall on the grass, are swallowed by sheep, rabbits, cattle, &c., and may give rise to the disease known as "sturdy" or "turnsick." The ova develope into those cystic worms known as the "many-headed gid hydatid," which prefer to reside in the brain.

3. *T. marginata*.—Its cystic form is the long-necked bladder-worm found in the peritoneal sac of herbivores, especially sheep.

* Its occurrence *naturally* in the muscles of foxes is mentioned in the 'Allegemeinige Med. Cent. Zeitung.'

134 THE DISEASES OF THE DOG.

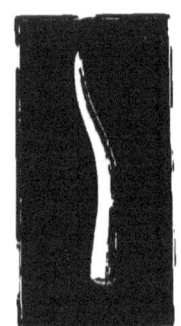

FIG. 37.—The "Mawworm."

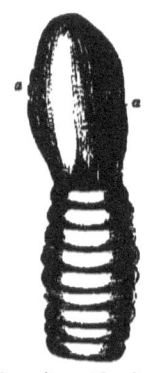

FIG. 37A.—Head of *Bothriocephalus latus*.

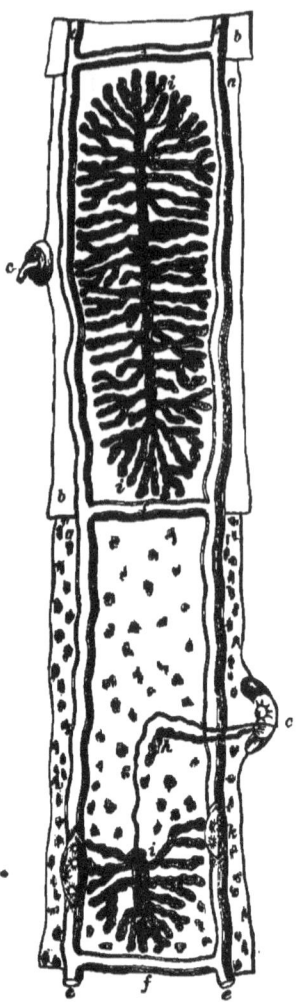

FIG. 37B.—*Tænia solium*, showing details of structure.

c. Generative orifice. e. Water vascular canals. g. Ovarian duct. h. Ovarian receptacle. i. Branched ovarium.

37, 37A, B) Parasites after STONEHENGE.

ON THE DISORDERS OF THE DIGESTIVE APPARATUS. 135

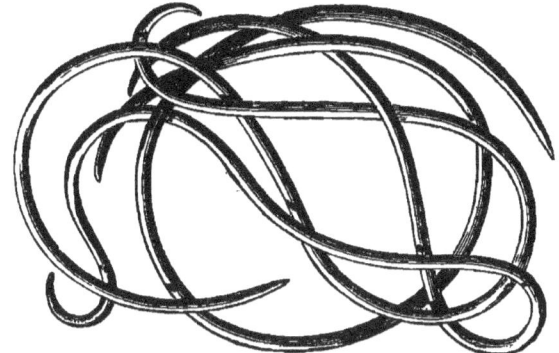

FIG. 38.—Ascarides.

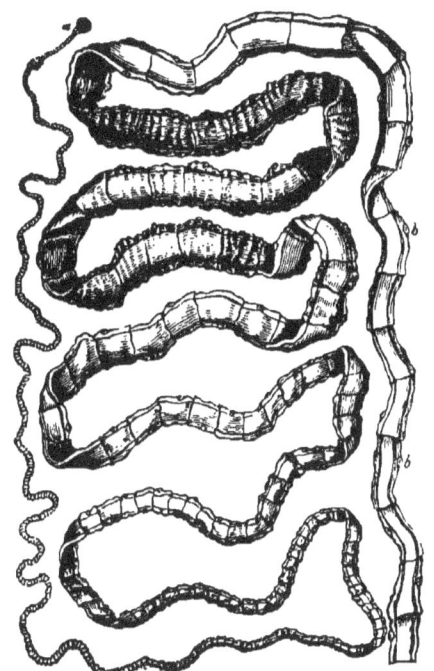

FIG. 39.—*Tænia solium.*
a. Head. *b.* Generative orifice.

(38 and 39) Parasites after STONEHENGE.

4. *T. echinococcus* is a very small tapeworm, but has a very large cystic form, which gives rise to true hydatids in man and other animals. These frequent especially the liver and lungs, and sometimes attain the size of a cricket ball, and by accidental rupture cause death.

5. *T. serrata* has, as its larval form, *Cysticercus pisiformis* of the hare and rabbit. The adult tapeworm is, therefore, said to be most frequent in harriers and greyhounds.*

Our efforts for lessening the number of tapeworms must comprise destruction of the fæces of affected animals, also of the hydatid-infested organs of herbivora, also of the tapeworms which are obtained on post-mortem examination or expelled as the result of medicinal treatment. As a tæniafuge the best agent decidedly for ordinary use in canine practice is areca nut in doses of from half a drachm to two drachms according to the size of the patient. It should be combined with a cathartic. Oil of turpentine is always available and can be freely utilised if combined with bland oil of twice or thrice its bulk, about three fluid drachms being the maximum dose ; it acts promptly and effectually. Vermifuges should always be followed by vegetable and mineral tonics as soon as the action of the accompanying cathartic has passed of. We need scarcely add that with the means already at our disposal we no longer deem it right to give the so-called mechanical vermifuges, liquid mercury, powdered glass, cowhage, or tin filings ; where collections of worms give rise to intestinal obstruction, as is occasionally the case, the nature of the impaction will probably not be discovered until after death.

Anacker, of Berne, writing to Der Thierarzt, 1875, points out the frequency of disease from worms penetrating the intestines, especially Ascarides which have a horny mouth, in some cases furnished with teeth. Agglomeration of these worms frequently causes fatality of dogs and cats, by suction giving rise to minute red ulcers and true catarrhal enteritis ; *Tænia crassicollis* also acts thus in the

---

* *Bothriocephalus latus*, a form of tapeworm found in the dog and man, is of little clinical importance ; nor is *Tænia literata* important, but it must be noted as having been found in the small intestines of the dog and cat.

cat. *Holostoma alatum*, a fluke, occasionally is found in the stomach and intestine of the dog. *Cheiracanthus* occurs in the stomach of the dog ('Veterinarian,' 1875, p. 115).

APPENDIX I.—THE PERITONEUM.

The peritoneum of the dog is not liable to inflammation as a result of surgical operations, as physiologists have amply proved, and so also have veterinary surgeons in the operation of LAPAROTOMY. Thus Felizet, of Elbœuf (*vide* 'Journal de Méd. Vét.,' 1853, p. 40), relates several cases of recovery after operation on the dog for removal of concretions from the intestines, and numerous successful cases of the Cæsarean operation on the bitch are now on record, *vide*, for example, 'Annales de Méd. Vét.,' 1878, p. 241, where five are mentioned. Yet the experience of canine pathologists tends to the conclusion that the peritoneum of the dog is rather liable to inflammation from non-surgical causes, especially to the chronic form of the disorder.

PERITONITIS when acute is difficult to distinguish from enteritis, indeed it generally accompanies the latter. Fever runs high, and the animal utters sharp cries, especially when handled; the breathing is difficult, and obstinate constipation is present. The dog is extremely restless and cannot lie down with comfort. In the chronic and more frequent form the symptoms are similar but less marked, the belly is tucked up, hard, and painful on pressure, the animal endeavours to hide itself and becomes much emaciated, and the symptoms of dropsy of the belly supervene, as also may be the case in the more acute form, in which, however, gangrenous changes may carry off the patient. This disease generally results from external injury or exposure to cold. In the latter case it is probably rheumatic, which is considered the most frequent form of peritonitis in the dog. The inflammation is usually diffused, local patches of inflammation of the serous membrane of the belly only occurring in consequence of injury or in association with some morbid growth in connection with some abdominal organ.

Treatment consists in the application of fomentations to the belly, or mild stimulation may be of use in the earlier stages, also the application of leeches may give immediate relief. It is recognised that the exhibition of even the mildest purgatives is not admissible in these cases, and reliance should be placed on full doses of sedatives such as digitalis, aconite, and especially opium. The latter to be given in the crude form to lessen pain.

ASCITES is often described as chronic peritonitis, but it may be present without inflammation of the lining membrane of the belly. It is more frequent as a non-specific disorder in the dog than in any other of our domesticated mammals. It is generally due to derangement of the liver, but occurs sometimes as a result of simple debility especially the persistent form of anæmia which follows as a complication of long-standing asthma or chronic skin disease. Whitworth, in an article contributed to the 'Veterinary Journal,' vol. xi, p. 394, attributes it generally to cirrhotic disease of liver, but ascites more generally in the dog is due to fatty or malignant change of that organ. The disease is seen in young dogs as a result of exposure of weak animals to cold and damp. *Symptoms*.—In addition to those of the disease on which it depends, we find enlargement of the belly, a rough coat with loose hair, frequent vomition, dulness and increasing marasmus, the visible mucous membranes pale; some indigestion is usually present, and subacute fever, a symptomatic cough, and hurried breathing. The patient generally suffers from intolerable thirst. As the disease advances general œdema sets in and the fatal result may be brought about by suffocation. *Diagnosis*.—This disorder must be carefully distinguished from other states, normal and abnormal, which lead to pendulous and enlarged belly. In ascites, the fluid gravitates to the lower part and gives the sides a flattened appearance; although the animal is pot-bellied he is hollow in the flanks; by alteration in the position the shape of the belly may be changed, also on percussion and succussion the fluctuation of fluid is detectable. In pregnancy the fœtus can be felt on manipulation, and the teats begin to enlarge and the mammary gland to swell; in obesity the body in general is fat and the shape does not alter with the position of the animal, the belly is rounded at the flank as well as at the sides, and no fluctuation detectable; in liver or spleen enlargement there is an absence of fluctuation, and usually a tumour may be felt in the anterior part of the belly. A case of enlarged spleen lying along the floor of the belly and very soft, is difficult to distinguish from one of ascites. In the latter disease, however, the skin seems tense, the hair is loose, the breathing disturbed, and in the more advanced cases the œdema sets in below the jaw and in the limbs and is very distinctive.

Treatment.—Generally requires to be tonic; vegetable bitters are useful. Digitalis is especially valuable and iodide of iron in small doses. Laxatives, such as calomel and aloes, are advocated by some practitioners, but they require to be administered with the greatest care and judgment. Cod-liver oil as a nutritive and very mild laxative is often followed by great benefit. The operation of TAPPING THE BELLY, *Paracentesis abdominis*, performed with the trochar and cannula (under the usual precautions) at the linea alba against the umbilicus affords some hope of relief where organic disease of the liver and spleen is absent, but it may be required several times to relieve the dyspnœa. *After-treatment* for the operation consists in support of the belly by means of a bandage. It is considered that in the dog, contrary to what is observed in man, all the fluid may be removed at one time without damage.

140 THE DISEASES OF THE DOG.

Appendix II—THE LIVER, PANCREAS, AND SPLEEN, &c.

THE liver of the dog is large, well developed, and much lobulated; it has but a thin and delicate Glisson's capsule,

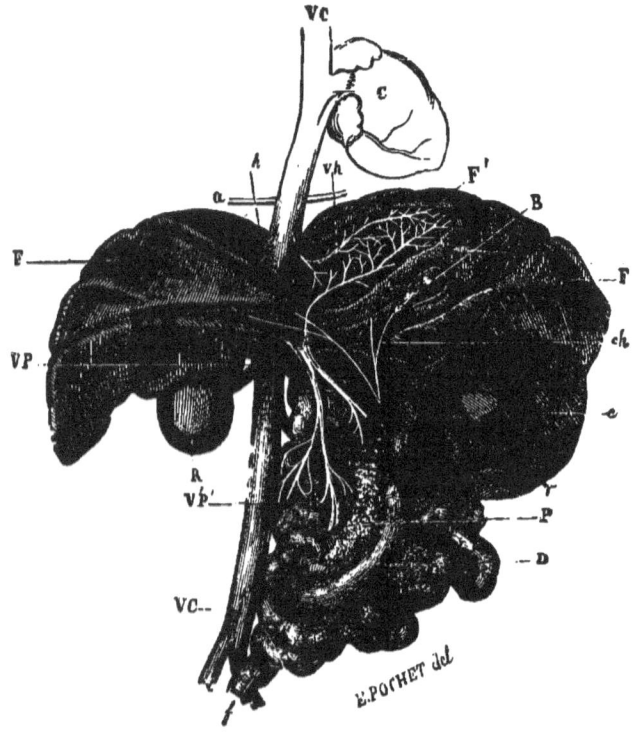

FIG. 40.—Liver, &c., from FLEMING's translation of CHAUVEAU's Anatomy.
  V.P. Vena portæ. V.C. Venæ cavæ. B. Gall-bladder. P. Pancreas.
  e. Stomach. D. Duodenum. R. Kidney. F. Lobes of liver.

and thus, even for its size, represents considerable secreting power; its gall-bladder is well developed, and the common duct receives a small branch from the pancreas before terminating at the bowel at a varying distance from the stomach (one to four inches). The gall-bladder is almost buried in the substance of the liver when the lobes lie in their normal position. The bile of the dog, as of other carnivora, is yellow, it is remarkable for the fact that the whole of its bilin consists of taurocholate.

The amount of bile secreted by a dog in twenty-four hours is from six to twelve drachms. Haller, from his experiments, placed the average amount secreted at twelve and a half drachms. The rate of secretion will depend upon the digestion; while the animal is fasting no bile is formed, but within a few minutes of giving food the bile is secreted freely, and continues until digestion is finished.

Schwann's experiments made on dogs to determine the uses of the bile, showed that if a fistula was established between the gall-bladder and skin, and the common duct tied so that the whole amount of bile secreted was poured out externally, that in those animals which survived the operation for any length of time, enfeebled nutrition, muscular weakness, falling off of the hair, &c., occurred; these symptoms were aggravated the longer the animal lived; death usually took place two or three weeks after the operation. In Blondlot's experiments a dog with a biliary fistula lived three months; he at first lost weight, then improved, but never regained his normal condition.

The liver of the dog is especially liable to disease, which generally assumes the form of chronic degeneration, but in tropical climates is not unfrequently acute. Diseases of the liver are in this, as in other species, characterised by jaundice, but when that distinctive symptom is not present, they are more or less obscure forms of indigestion with a tendency to anæmia. There can be no doubt that they very frequently remain entirely undetected during the life of the animal, and are often mistaken for other diseases, especially those of the stomach. If we consider the stimulating influence of flesh food on the liver, the largeness of the bile excretory apparatus of the dog, and the deficiency of exercise given to dogs of the fancy breeds, we will not be surprised to find the liver a frequent seat of disease in canine animals.

HEPATITIS in its *acute form* is common in India and other tropical countries; it also has been reported as frequent in the South of France. It is probably in most cases congestive, rather than true inflammatory disorder. Jaundice is a prominent symptom; the patient becomes very dull, restless, and seeks a dark, quiet place; much thirst is present; frequent vomition of a material consisting mainly of bile occurs, but the act of expulsion seems to be not very painful. Pressure on the right side over the liver causes acute pain, and the belly is sometimes enlarged in consequence of the swelling of that organ. Breathing is quick and panting; cough may be present. The patient eats nothing, his mouth is foul, and the gums congested; generally the fæces are dry and pale coloured, but in some cases the bowels are rather loose. Occasionally, what Blaine terms "bilious inflammation of the bowels" sets in, there being much abdominal pain and a copious expulsion of bile in the frequent vomits and alvine evacuations. This proves very exhausting and may carry off the animal, the bowels after death being found inflamed probably by the acridity of the bile; but we are warned to distinguish in diagnosis between it and irritant poisoning by the animal being more thirsty in the latter case and passing blood intermingled with the black ejecta from the bowels. The acute symptoms sometimes subside gradually and are replaced by those indicative of *chronic* liver disorder; in other cases symptoms of cerebral disturbance may precede death, or paralysis occur; generally increasing pallor of visible membranes, and marked coldness of the mouth precede death. It having been found that this disorder may be mistaken for pleuro-pneumonia or enteritis, Blaine points out that there is less coldness of and watery discharge from the nose and mouth than in the former disease, and less pain on pressure, tension, and heat of the belly, also less prostration of strength than in the latter.* *Treatment.*—Certainly a moderate bleeding, when promptly resorted to, is the best means of dealing with an acute case, and its action may be materially assisted by mustard plasters over the liver and use of the warm bath. Leeches to the side over the liver have been found of benefit. The greatest care should be taken to avoid exposure to cold after removal from the bath, the patient being carefully wrapped up in a blanket. As for internal agents, we may anticipate most benefit from Epsom salts, nitre, and sal ammoniac, in small doses thrice a day.† Antimony and mercurial compounds must be avoided, the former on account of their influence on the stomach and the latter as likely to hyperstimulate the liver. Frequent small doses of dilute vinegar constitute an excellent domestic remedy in these cases, and on recovery the animal will require most careful attention to dieting.

CHRONIC HEPATITIS also is generally congestive rather than due to inflammation. It is probably one of the most frequent disorders of the dog, and may be traced to causes such as when they act powerfully and simultaneously produce acute inflammation. These are generally insidious in their effects, gradually producing congestion of the liver and degenerative changes of its component elements. Exposure to cold and damp, especially in a malarious climate, may cause acute congestion in a liver predisposed by a long course of high feeding uncounterbalanced by sufficient exercise. Exposure for a long time to the relaxing effects of heat, abuse of medicines which stimulate the liver, sudden immersion in water when the animal is very hot, injury from violence over the seat of the organ, are causes of disorder. In England want of exercise, over-feeding, and the moistness of the climate are the main causes of chronic liver disorder, whereas in India it principally results also from malaria and prolonged high external temperature.

* Mayhew has recorded a case of liver abscess in a setter from which more than two gallons of pus of a watery character was extracted.

† Williams advocates elaterium for the relief of liver congestion in dogs, it causes watery stools.

The *Symptoms* are at first jaundice of a subacute character, constant dulness, frequent vomition, unthrifty coat, swollen right side of the belly, persistent thirst, indigestion, flatulence, and extreme irregularity of the bowels. The patient eats but little, wastes away rapidly, his belly becomes pendulous, but on manipulation this is found not due to dropsy; piles are a common result of pressure of the swollen liver on the large veins passing through it. It has been observed that the wasting of the animal often occurs suddenly after it has been extremely fat, its skin becomes much disordered, rough, harsh, and scabby. Asthma and splenic disorders have been noted as not infrequent accompaniments. The form of distemper in which the liver is principally affected must not be taken

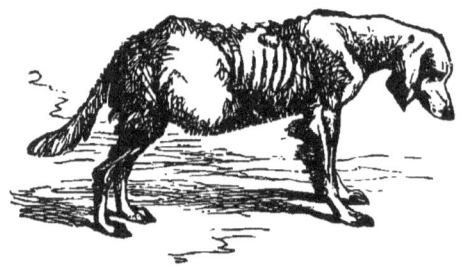

Fig. 41.—Liver disorder (MAYHEW).

as primary liver disease, although occasionally it induces such changes of the organ as to render it unfit to perform its duties. *Treatment* of chronic disorder of the liver comprises careful regulation of the bowels by the use of salines, especially Epsom salts combined with sal ammoniac and nitre; small doses of calomel and podophyllin are often beneficial to arouse the torpid organ to action. Aloes also may be given and the mineral acids in small doses, especially the hydrochloric, are likely to prove beneficial. Occasional stimulation of the skin of the right hypochondrium, such as by painting it with tincture of iodine, as advocated by Hill, may be resorted to. Careful regulation of diet and exercise will prove more useful than medicine, but, with Mayhew, we must urge that "the food must not suddenly be reduced to starvation point. . . . The structures have been so much changed that medicine cannot be expected to restore them. The pet may be saved to its indulgent mistress, and again perhaps exhibit all the charms for which it was ever prized; but the sporting dog will never be made capable of doing work, and certainly it is not to be selected to breed from after it has sustained an attack of hepatitis."

DEGENERATIONS OF THE LIVER in carnivora generally assume the fatty form, the organ being enlarged and softened. Sometimes the enlargement is extreme and detectable with the greatest facility, and the liver is practically a mass of fat, the result of both true fatty degeneration and of infiltration. Magendie, the illustrious physiologist, fed a dog on fresh butter for sixty-eight days; it became remarkably fat, but died ultimately of inanition. Throughout the course of the experiment the animal smelt strongly of butyric acid, and its hair was greasy. The liver was very fatty, "and, on analysis, it was found to contain a very large quantity of stearine, but little or no oleine; it had acted as a kind of filter for the butter" (Budd). Other dogs fed wholly on fat became very fat but anæmic. We see similar experiments involuntarily performed by dog-owners around us on every side daily; pampered, highly-fed pets become sluggish in their movements, enormously fat, anæmic, irregular in the bowels, and big in the belly. They may succumb to coexistent fatty degeneration of the heart, or suddenly lose flesh and show all the signs of chronic hepatitis. A gradual alteration of the diet and increase of the amount of exercise taken may be tried when fatty liver is diagnosed. A small amount of fresh liver should be given occasionally in the food. Medicinally, benefit may result from small doses of chlorate of potash given daily for a long time. Cirrhosis, amyloid change, and other degenerations of the liver are not often seen in dogs. *Rupture of the liver* has been recorded only as a result of injury.

MALIGNANT DISEASE OF THE LIVER is more frequent in carnivora than in other lower animals and generally assumes the form of spindle-celled sarcoma. The liver is seldom the only abdominal organ affected, the spleen, mesentery, and omentum being also the seat of yellowish-grey nodulated tumours. The patients thus affected are generally old and worn out by the disease, and their destruction is evidently the most advisable course to adopt.

PARASITIC DISEASE of the liver of the dog has been described by Dr. Lewis, of Calcutta. He found flukes, *Distoma conjunctum*, frequent in the bile-ducts of pariahs. Dr. Cobbold also found them in the American red fox. The latter observation was made about in 1860; the para-

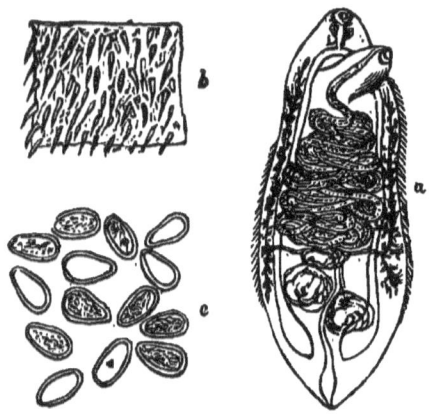

FIG. 42.—*Distoma conjunctum*, after COBBOLD.
(a) The parasite. (b) Spines on a portion of its integument. (c) Ova.

sites had given rise to "inflammation and the formation of small cysts or abscesses, apparently causing the death of the host." Cystic parasites are remarkably infrequent in or on the liver of the dog. Reiman* has observed and described invasion of the liver and other organs of the dog by echinococci. Mather observed small nematodes (*Filaria hepatica*) in the liver-ducts and substance, as well as in cysts within the walls of the intestines. *Ectopia hepatis* has been also observed in canine patients.

* 'Deut. Zelt. f. Thiermed. u. Verg. Path.,' B. 11, p. 81.

THE EXCRETORY APPARATUS OF THE LIVER.—The dog is the animal most frequently used by physiologists for obtaining bile in a perfectly fresh state. The non-liability of the dog to traumatic peritonitis, and the facility of access to his bile-duct accounts for his usually being selected for the production of a *biliary fistula*. Gamgee thus describes the operation : " An incision three or four inches long is made in the linea alba, commencing at the xiphoid cartilage, and the peritoneum having been carefully divided the liver is raised, when the gall-bladder comes into view. This having been seized with a pair of forceps and drawn to the surface, the cystic and hepatic ducts are seen joining to form the common bile-duct, which is easily seen entering the duodenum. Two ligatures are then passed around this duct, one being placed as near the gut as possible, the other near the origin of the duct. The portion between the two ligatures is cut out. The gallbladder is now fixed to the anterior part of the wound by means of metallic sutures, and then opened sufficiently to admit the little finger. The rest of the wound is closed by metallic sutures ; the quill suture is, perhaps, the best. Care must be taken to bring the wound in the muscles together before sewing up that of the skin. After the operation a wide roller is passed round the belly of the dog, a hole being made in it to allow the escape of the bile. If matters proceed satisfactorily the wound in the abdominal wall heals, except where the opening in the gall-bladder becomes adherent."

BILIARY CALCULI are not rare in the dog ; they vary in consistence from inspissated bile masses to hard concretions. They prove of importance either as causing jaundice by entering the duct and obstructing it or else by the acute pain which occurs during their passage. When jaundiced animals suddenly manifest acute pain by extreme violence and loud cries it is generally due to passage of gall-stones. This must be, encouraged and rendered less painful by warm baths and administration of opiates, and immediate relief, not only of the pain but also of any jaundice associated with it, will follow expulsion of the stones. They are generally present in numbers, so the pain is apt to recur. Administration of occasional doses of podophyllin or calomel will be useful to prevent stagnation of bile in the gall-bladder and duct, and its consequent inspissation.

The PANCREAS of the dog is large and well developed, being much more compact and well defined than that of the horse. It is V-shaped and pours its secretion through two main ducts into the bowel, one of which blends with

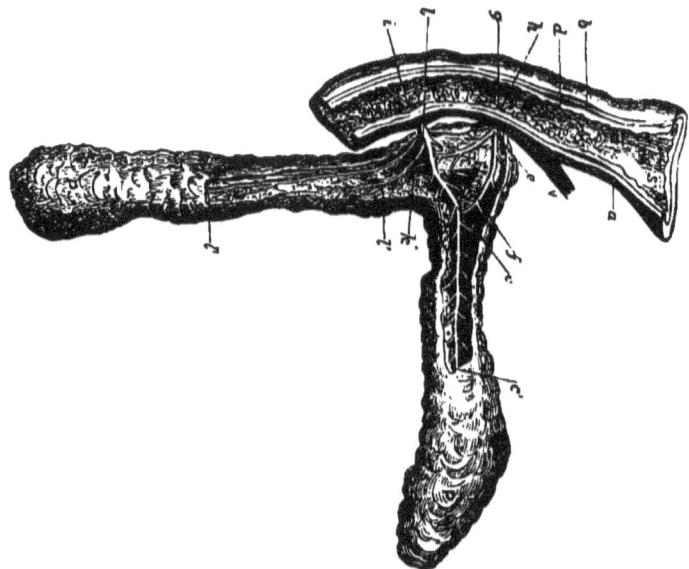

FIG. 43.—Pancreas, after GAMGEE.

a, b, d. Coats of the bowel. s. Cavity of duodenum. v. Bile-duct. c, e, f, c', k, l'. Ducts of pancreas. P. Pancreas lobes. i, l, h, g. Openings of ducts into duodenum.

the common bile-duct. The secretion from the dog has been obtained by tying a tube in the duct as exposed by laparotomy, but "it is quite impossible to establish a permanent pancreatic fistula like a permanent hepatic or gastric fistula, for the tube falls out in the course of two or three days, and the wound healing up, the animal gradually recovers" (Gamgee). This organ has not been recognised as the seat of disorder in the dog, except that in 1850 M. Bernard exhibited before the Société de Biologie a dog in which a pancreatic fistula had been made, but which died in a state of extreme emaciation. It was found that *the pancreas had completely disappeared*; it was believed it had been digested by the bile ('Gaz. Méd.,' 9th March, 1850).

The SPLEEN is well developed and less markedly sickle-shaped than in the horse. Evidence tends to show that it is much more frequently diseased in carnivora than herbivora, and numerous cases are on record showing the nature and phenomena of splenic disorder in the dog. These cases are seldom recognised ante mortem, being mistaken for liver derangement. The various British authors on canine pathology speak of SPLENITIS, but apparently without distinct evidence as to the exact pathological state to be dealt with. Blaine summarises his views on this subject by saying, " Whenever a dog has been unthrifty in his coat, and irregular in his evacuations, I have almost invariably found that both the liver and spleen of the animal were more or less indurated and swollen, particularly the latter." This state results from long confinement, and the animal being gorged with flesh; the patient becomes unthrifty in the coat, much emaciated, and loose in his stools; he husks and vomits frequently; the evacuations are yellow and frothy, or at times constipation is present; there is tumour at the left side of the front of the belly, which is painful on pressure, so the dog cries when moved; he is feverish and the visible mucous membranes pale. These symptoms, generally described as those of splenitis, should be considered as indicative of chronic spleen disorder of one of the forms to be described immediately. They are practically incurable. Laparotomy for their removal does not generally prove successful because the spleen is seldom the only organ diseased, the liver (as sufficiently indicated by the above enumerated symptoms) and the mesenteric glands being usually involved; also we cannot often detect spleen disease in its earliest and uncomplicated stages and it not unfrequently is the manifestation of some systemic disorder. Thus it is found in leukæmia, a disease not infrequent in the dog, and in malarious fevers.

Excision of the Spleen is an operation which is not unfrequently performed for physiological inquiries, and carnivora are capable of resisting the constitutional effects of removal of this large organ, probably by compensatory increase of other hæmatogenic organs, also they are very tolerant of the operation for its ablation. This nonessentiality of the spleen accounts for its being capable of undergoing extensive disease changes without material interference with the animal's health. Medicinal treatment is not likely to be effectual, although the influence of iodine and tonic doses continued for a long time may be tried, and the bowels kept open by aloes and calomel. As the organ increases in size (and it sometimes attains enormous proportions) it much encroaches on the space in the belly occupied by the bowels, and causes disturbance of them.

HÆMORRHAGIC TUMOURS of the spleen are often found in the dog; generally they are of some standing as denoted by the conditions of successive clots. Adams, of Oossoor, relates* an instance in which the organ was of enormous size (21½ in. long and 9 inches broad; weight 6 lbs.) and quite a jelly-like mass lying along the whole floor of the belly. The patient was an Australian deerhound and died from *rupture of the organ,* where it lay against the pelvis. The rupture Mr. Adams considered due to very slight exertion, the disease of the spleen to cachexia induced by the change of climate from Australia to India. In my experience, these cases are always found in large dogs; they generally involve only part of the spleen; they usually prove fatal by rupture. They seem non-malignant in nature. I find three mentioned in my notebook; one was a true hæmorrhagic tumour in a mastiff bitch in a state of chronic anæmia, another in a retriever dog, also anæmic; in each case the spleen was detectable as en-

* 'Veterinary Journal,' xx, p. 250.

larged before death and bulged out behind the ribs on the left side. The third patient was a large boarhound treated at the Royal Veterinary College, London. On admission he was in f..ir condition, but he fell away in flesh and looked bad in his coat. The spleen was found of enormous size and gorged with blood after death, which was considered as due to *splenic apoplexy*, not the form of anthrax known under that name, however.

Sarcomatous Growth in, and other Malignant Disease of the Spleen of the Dog is not rare. The case by Gowing, of Camden Town,* is a good example of this disease. In leukæmia and anthrax the spleen is often the principal seat of lesions detected post mortem.

Diseases of the other Ductless Glands.—The THYROID BODY is well developed in dogs and liable to enlargement, either of an acute or chronic character. BRONCHOCELE or GOITRE is specially frequent in carnivora among quadrupeds, and differs in some very important respects from the same disease in man. Thus it is not endemic and is often very acute. It can generally be associated with starvation and dirt, although it is not unfrequent in newly-born pups, and as often several in a litter suffer from it, and it is generally an accompaniment of rickets or deformities, it is considered hereditary, although possibly rather due to malnutrition of the female parent during utero-gestation. It especially occurs in certain breeds, pugs being most liable to it. They have large glands in the throat (vulgarly called "*kernels*") while young, and the enlargement decreases in proportion to growth in the majority of cases or readily yields to absorbent treatment, external and internal. It has been noted, however, that the swelling of the glands is periodically recurrent, and so an apparently favorable result of treatment may prove deceptive. Youatt tells us "there is a breed of the Blenheim spaniel in which this periodical goitre is very remarkable; the slightest cold is accompanied by enlargement of the thyroid gland, but the swelling altogether disappears in the course of a fortnight." As a rule

* 'Veterinary Journal,' x, p. 385.

painting the part, after removal of the hair, with tincture of iodine, and the internal administration of iodine in half-grain doses morning and evening will permanently reduce the enlargement. The introduction of setons, excision of the glands, blistering, and other heroic methods should not be resorted to. In acute cases, as described by Youatt, the sudden enlargement of the thyroid is considerable, and pressure is brought about on the jugulars, trachea, and œsophagus, which are all more or less obstructed, and suffocation may result. The patient sleeps much, is dull, and may die quietly; symptoms probably the result of *jugular* obstruction. In some cases suppuration occurs, and very extensive ulceration as a sequela; these are probably scrofulous in their nature, and generally prove incurable.

The THYMUS BODY is large in puppies, and slow to disappear. It is entirely confined to the anterior mediastinum, and there is no record to hand of it being diseased in carnivora.

CHAPTER VII.—THE URINARY APPARATUS.

THE kidneys of our domesticated carnivora are rounded and reniform, unlobulated, and with a single elongated papilla projecting into the central cavity of each. The bladder has muscular walls of great thickness, so that the urine is expelled with considerable force. It also is got rid of frequently, is of a lighter colour and stronger odour than that of herbivora, and contains no hippuric acid. The urinary apparatus of the dog is rather liable to calculous concretions, and ALBUMINOUS NEPHRITIS, true Bright's disease, has been found in him, and is probably more frequent than is generally supposed. Prof. Axe, of the London School, exhibited a case of this disorder before the Central Veterinary Society, and described the granular degeneration, cystic formations (from retention), fatty change, and other conditions characteristic of the disease, which he found as well developed in the kidney of the dog as of man. Mathis found in a case of this disease in the dog, arteritis and periarteritis, sclerosis, atrophy, and degeneration of the kidneys. The patient was destroyed after a period of increasing debility following endocarditis ; constipation, thirst, profuse urination, capricious appetite, laziness, cries when moved, and inclination to keep constantly near the fire were the principal symptoms in this case ('Jnl. de Méd. Vét. et de Zoot.'). The detection of albumen in the urine is not an absolute proof of the presence of this derangement, for it may depend on the nature of the food. When in cases of obscure marasmus the boiling and nitric tests show albumen present, Bright's disease of one or both of the kidneys may be suspected and the animal considered incurable, although small doses of iodide of iron and cod-liver oil may be resorted to for prolonging his life if he be a favourite. NEPHRITIS or RENITIS is not frequent except as a result of injury, as when a carriage passes over the loins. Thanks to the thickness of both supra- and sub-lumbar muscles of the dog this accident often causes no serious damage, but with a heavy vehicle moving at a slow pace the loin bones may be crushed and the kidneys are liable to be bruised. An abscess may form in the injured organ or it may undergo such disorganization as to become totally absorbed, for sometimes on post-mortem examination of the dog but one kidney, a large one, is found. This may also result from congenital irregularity. Calculi in the kidney cause suppuration and sometimes extensive removal of its glandular substance by gradual absorption. It is said that the imprudent use of aphrodisiacs (Youatt) and cantharides blister absorbed from the surface or licked by the patient (Hill) cause this disorder. Exposure to inclement weather and retention of urine are also advanced as causes. A patient affected with nephritis suffers from high fever, straddles in his gait, feels and shows acute pain when pressed over the loins, and moves about in a very uncomfortable way, constantly attempting to urinate. The fluid passed is scanty and high coloured and may contain pus or blood. Later, coma, insensibility, and frequent vomition sets in, the result of retention of urea in the blood. *Treatment* consists in keeping the animal quiet and administering opium and demulcent drinks. Opiate enemata are useful, and the loins should be stimulated, fomented, or poulticed, as the urgency of the symptoms seem to demand. Leeches have been applied to the loins with benefit.

RENAL CALCULUS is a concretion of which we have numerous cases on record. One or both kidneys may be occupied and have undergone enlargement (with dilatation of the pelvis) and inflammatory changes. The chemical composition of the calculi, which are usually numerous, has been found to be urate of ammonia and phosphate with oxalate of lime. The symptoms vary; at times they are indicative of very acute renal irritation and inflammation, with great pain in voiding fæces; at other times the patient suffers but little irritation. There can be no doubt that many small calculi form and pass from the kidney without causing the animal any inconvenience, but in the bladder they may become the nuclei of new concretions. The inflammation of the kidney must be treated, and especially opium given in quantity to allay pain, which also may be effected by use of warm water. Hill recommends mild diuretics and laxatives to encourage the descent of the calculi, also mucilaginous drinks and sharp exercise. These cases are not easy to diagnose; at most the presence of calculus is only shrewdly suspected in nephritis.

ATROPHY and HYPERTROPHY of the kidney are not unfrequently found and are not always disease. They seldom are detectable during life and also seldom cause inconvenience. HYDATIDS of this organ, mentioned by Blaine as being more frequent in the dog than in man, are probably merely *cysts of retention* due to blocking up of the tubuli uriniferi, either from Bright's disease or from simple concretions of urine salts and mucus in the tubuli uriniferi.

PARASITES.—*Eustrongylus gigas* has been found in the kidney of the dog. Its female has been observed over a yard in length and as large round as the little finger.

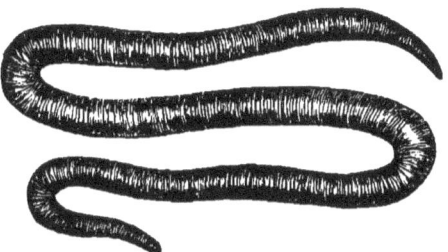

FIG. 44.—*Eustrongylus gigas*, after COBBOLD.

The URETER is occasionally blocked by impaction of escaping renal calculi; this is generally spasmodic and acutely painful, but the spasm ultimately yields, and the stone passes on into the bladder. Sometimes the ureters are chronically dilated, and they may contain sabulous matter.

CYSTITIS is generally of rare occurrence, but Blaine and Youatt have placed on record an epizooty of it observed by them in 1810. It is attributed when sporadic to prolonged retention of urine, irritation from calculi or parasites, and strangury induced by imprudent use of cantharides or turpentine, internally or externally. Mechanical injury is mentioned as a cause. Perhaps it most frequently results from obstruction to the passage of urine by abnormality of the prostate. The patient exhibits extreme restlessness and colicky pains; he constantly changes his posture and his hind limbs tremble; he is anxious and extremely irritable. Fever is present, and much pain is expressed on pressure of the walls of the belly, especially against the pelvis, towards which part the animal sometimes looks anxiously. Urine is passed *guttatim* or is suppressed, and the act or attempt at expulsion is painful. In more chronic cases the symptoms very closely resemble those of nephritis.

Treatment.—Relieve pain by hot baths and opiates, which means will also overcome spasm of the urethra; local bleeding by means of leeches to the perinæum is useful, as also are fomentations and emollient enemata. Mucilaginous and alkaline drinks may be given. The catheter should be passed to ensure the absence of retention or obstruction, which must be overcome if detected. The bowels in chronic cases should be constantly regulated, and exploration made to determine whether calculus is present or no.

CYSTIC CALCULUS must be considered as frequent in the dog, and cases are on record also in the bitch. Analysis has shown that these concretions are composed of triple phosphate and phosphate of lime. They vary much in size and external form, some being smooth and spherical, others spicular and irregular; naturally the latter are the source of the greatest amount of irritation. Generally more than one calculus is present, and the smaller ones and sabulous matter or gravel are passed periodically, and Gowing records that in one of his cases the latter became

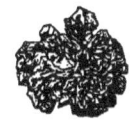 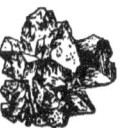

FIG. 45.—Cystic calculus, after MORTON.

deposited on the hair below the generative opening in a bitch. The urine varies in colour; sometimes it is red, and distinctly contains blood, in other cases it is yellow and thick from apparently pus, really urine crystals. The smaller breeds of dogs are most liable to calculi in the bladder, which are generally nucleated. Boerhaave produced one by the artificial introduction of a small rounded pebble, which acted as a centre of deposit in the course of a few months. With the symptoms of chronic cystitis we find in these cases a continuous flow of urine, and resulting excoriation. The current is uncertain, and

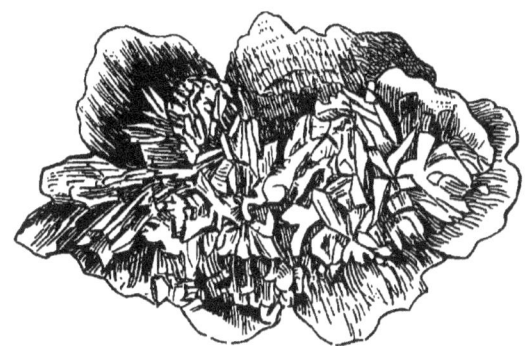

FIG. 46.—Cystic calculus, after MORTON.

may be suddenly suppressed, and the animal show much pain. In some cases there is detectable swelling in the perinæum in the male. Mayhew considers as diagnostic the animal finding a difficulty in going downstairs, having frequent fits of pain, " aud the point of the penis is protruded from the sheath, never being withdrawn." The leg is not raised to void the urine, but the creature strains violently when the act has either been accomplished, or there is no power to perform it. If the dog be taken on the knee, and one knowing the situation of the contents gently manipulates the abdomen, the body may be felt within the bladder, which will mostly be contracted and empty. A very interesting case of calculus in the bladder was recorded by Professor Morton, and the specimen may be seen in the museum of the London School. The stone practically fills the viscus, and could easily be felt during life. Mayhew frankly confesses that he has never performed LITHOTOMY on the dog, and he doubts whether we would find it practicable, considering the delicacy of the patient and the smallness of the parts to be operated on. Certainly but few successful cases are on record, but it has been amply proved as not beyond the power of the canine surgeon. Hill ('Veterinary Journal,' vol. xiii, p. 43) describes a successful performance of the operation, but subsequent death from peritonitis. The patient was a St. Bernard bitch ; 202 calculi, varying in size from that of a millet to a potato, were extracted ; the largest weighed three ounces, and the total mass weighed nine ounces ; they were perfectly smooth and white, and mostly triangular in form. The case was complicated by renal calculus. As usual in these cases, a stone had become fixed in the neck of the bladder and caused obstruction. Unless this obstruction is removed by operation, the bladder becomes mortified and the patient dies. The operation presents no special features when performed on the dog or bitch. Youatt informs us that occasionally a large calculus in the bladder is broken down by the forcible compression exerted on it by the muscular coat. This is a remarkable instance of *natural lithotrity*, an operation which is seldom needed in artificial removal because the calculi are usually small and numerous.

RUPTURE OF THE BLADDER occurs as the culmination of obstruction of the urethral passage in cases of diseased prostate. Sometimes, also, it follows unrelieved urethral obstruction by calculus. After the animal has for some time passed urine only drop by drop, and has seemed disinclined to move, he shows the symptoms above enumerated as indicative of acute cystitis ; these are succeeded by evident collapse, and the patient soon dies quietly. A bloody fluid is found in the belly post mortem, the peritoneum is congested, and the bladder (especially its mucous membrane) inflamed ; the walls are found more or less rent. This lesion is, of course, incurable.

CYSTIC HERNIA is not rare, especially in the bitch, for the neck of the bladder is rather long. It may be inguinal, femoral, or ventral. The symptoms are not generally acute, and the bladder is usually with other organs in the sac.

Stricture of the Neck of the Bladder and *eversion of that organ* have not, to my knowledge, been recorded in canine patients.

ABNORMAL URINATION occurs as an indication of disorder of the urinary apparatus. *Retention of urine* is found in urethral spasm or stricture, also in cases of prostatic disease and impacted calculus ; it is also seen in advanced debility and paralysis, and the distension of the bladder may be detected by manipulation of the belly. It must not been confounded with *suppression of urine,* the complete cessation of urine production indicative of inflammatory disease of both kidneys, or *scantiness of urine* as found in all fevers, and when one kidney only is inflamed. *Strangury* is the painful expulsion of urine *guttatim,* and not unfrequently that fluid is found intermingled with pus or blood. It occurs in renitis, also in cystitis, and partial obstruction of the urinary passage. *Incontinence of urine* occurs specially in bitches in consequence of cystic calculus or disease of the urino-genital passages. The constant dribbling away of urine causes excoriation of the skin over which it trickles. It has been known to temporarily result from prolonged retention of urine in a dog of good habits shut up in a room for a long time (Youatt). Tonics sufficed to check it in the case recorded.

PARALYSIS OF THE BLADDER results from prolonged retention and over-distension, but with rest the organ generally regains its tone. In some nervous disorders, especially apoplexy and injuries to the spinal cord, the paralysis persists, and small doses of nux vomica may be required. In cases of retention of urine the *catheter must be passed*. To perform this a human catheter of gum elastic is required, ranging from No. 1 to No. 5, according to the size of the animal; larger dogs even require Nos. 6, 7, and 8. The dog must be placed on its side and the penis drawn out, and then the catheter, without its wire and well lubricated with oil, is inserted into the urinary meatus and passed along the canal. The instrument meets with some obstruction at the osseous portion of the canal, but with care, patience, and delicacy of manipulation may be got beyond this. It is directed by the hand round the pubio-ischial arch, and then gradually passed to the bladder. Mayhew, who carefully describes this operation, warns us to immediately withdraw the catheter when the urine, instead of flowing in gentle slow stream, is ejected in jerks with force, "lest the bladder, energetically contracting upon it, should cause the point to pierce the sides of the viscus." This operation often needs repetition.

Profuse staling is seldom seen in the dog. The constant expulsion of a little urine by these animals when excited, or on starting for a run, is so familiar a phenomenon that it can never be mistaken for disease. Abuse of diuretics, and, it is said, bad food, may induce this derangement.

The *healthy urine of the dog* differs from that of vegetable feeders in the absence of hippuric acid, in its clear consistency, bright yellow colour and strong odour. Oxalic and uric calculi are more frequent in the dog than in herbivora. *Hæmaturia* is found in acute inflammations of the kidneys or bladder or as a result of injury, either external or caused by calculi. It is important to determine from what part of the urinary apparatus the hæmorrhage comes, and, this having been determined, astringent and styptic means may be adopted. Mayhew has found tincture of cantharides, 3 minims to water 2 oz., useful in these cases. In renal hæmorrhage the blood is passed as small worm-like clots diffused through the urine; in vesical hæmorrhage after expulsion of urine a flow of blood occurs; in urethral bleeding the blood, uncoagulated, trickles from the urethra without expulsive effort. The dark urine of hepatic and some blood disorders must not be considered bloody. DIABETES MELLITUS has been studied at the University of Naples by Prof. Ferraro. He finds that the disease occurs naturally in dogs, and in causes, symptoms, and treatment resembles the same disorder in man ('Il Morgagni,' 1885). *Urine with copious sediment* may contain excess of mucus, pus, sabulous matter, or gravel. In cases of doubt a little of the sediment may be put under the microscope, but that is usually superfluous. The passage of gravel is generally an indication of a tendency to the formation of urinary calculi, if not of their actual presence. To restrict the deposit, Mayhew recommends a strictly vegetable diet, doses of ether and laudanum both by mouth and injection; hyoscyamus and balsams, and sometimes cubebs or other peppers, and cantharides.

PROSTATIC DISEASE is so frequent in the dog that the casual manner in which it is noticed by authors on canine pathology is somewhat surprising. Youatt mentions a case of rupture of the bladder due to it, but without recognising what organ was "on the neck of the bladder the size of a goose's egg and almost filling the cavity of the pelvis; on cutting into it, more than 2 oz. of the pus escaped." Simonds* records a chronic case of gradual increase in size of the organ bringing about mechanical obstruction to the passage of urine. Mannington, of Brighton, was called to see a thirteen-year-old spaniel which for six months had shown a rapid increase in the size of the belly without impairment of the general health, and had been noticed latterly to urinate frequently. There was found immense enlargement and tenseness of the belly, especially at the sides; incessant attempts to

* 'Trans. V. M. A.,' 1840-41, p. 57.

void the urine were made and it was sometimes passed in small quantities. General marasmus, laboured breathing, disinclination to move, and pallid visible mucous membranes were the other symptoms. The belly was tapped, and about a pint of sero-sanguineous fluid trickled away slowly; the dog bore the operation well, but it had little effect in reducing the size of the abdomen, which now felt as if its contents were quite solid. The patient was given diffusible stimulants, but gradually sank and died nine hours after the operation. A tumour, the prostate in an enlarged state, was found hanging from the pubic region to the inferior part of the abdomen. It weighed 10½ lbs., whereas the rest of the carcass weighed only 15¼ lbs. ('Veterinary Record,' iii, 13th October, 1847). MacGillivray, of Banff, found prostatic disease in a large retriever dog which had been passing blood and matter in his urine. Progressive marasmus, stiffness and unwillingness to move, pain in passing urine, which act he performed every time he was taken from the kennel (and the flow of which ended in the passage of a couple of teaspoonfuls of very thin fluid pus, the last of which was tinged with blood), and a very disagreeable smell were the most prominent symptoms. Obstruction to passage of the catheter was also observed. The patient was treated with balsam of capivi and solutions of lunar caustic injected into the urethra. Severe rigors and heart-rending cries preceded death, which occurred about three weeks after the animal was first seen. Autopsy showed the prostate gland thrice its normal size, quite engorged with thin, purulent fluid of a most offensive odour. The bladder was half full of pus, and its mucous coat much thickened.* The above typical cases, from among a number recorded, illustrate the symptoms induced by this important lesion. Prostatic disease is so seldom seen in the other patients of veterinary surgeons that it is generally when found in the dog recorded as "pelvic tumour." Under this name I have had two cases sent to me for exhibition at professional meetings. The tumefaction of

* 'Veterinary Journal,' vol. xiii.

the gland can generally be detected by a finger inserted into the rectum; the enlarged belly, pelvic tumour, sometimes bulging perinæum, also obstruction to passage of the catheter and to expulsion of urine should suffice for detection of the abnormality. The age of the patient generally renders treatment inadvisable, as it can be but palliative. Incision into the tumour, or tapping the gland from the perinæum, may afford relief, but this disease is in dogs, as in old men, generally cystic, there being multiple small abscesses rather than one large collection of pus. The causes are obscure, but it is evidently a senile change and may be dependent on urethral inflammation, prostatitis, or other obstruction of the ducts of the gland, which is large and well developed in the dog and embraces the neck of the bladder on three sides. Cowper's glands, on the other hand, are absent. URETHRITIS occurs in the dog in association with BALANITIS (inflammation of the lining membrane of the prepuce) and POSTHITIS (inflammation of the mucous investment of the glans). It is caused by dirt, over-feeding, want of exercise, and debility, and is a frequent accompaniment of mange. It is generally seen in both indoor pets and watch-dogs, and, although commonly known as GONORRHŒA is not specific nor communicable. It cannot be traced to over-indulgence in sexual processes, but rather to deficiency in this respect. According as the external or internal parts are affected most, is the profuseness of the discharge. When the urethra is the main seat the glans is exposed, the penis being in a state of semi-erection almost constantly, and a small amount of fluid continually exudes from the opening. The animal licks the protruded part, and evidently suffers pain in the passage of urine. The discharge is either a thick mucus or purulent. When the external parts are the main seat of disorder, the prepuce is swollen and conceals the glans, phymosis to an extent being present. The prepuce contains much pus, which gradually oozes from the orifice and becomes dried on the hairs of the part, or flows profusely on pressure. There is obstruction to the passage of urine, the current of which is irregular. The animal resists exploration of the parts and retraction of the prepuce to expose the glans is a matter of some difficulty. In neglected cases ulcers form about the parts and a loathsome state of disorganisation ensues, the pus sometimes burrowing along the side of the penis and bursting out at intervals. *Treatment* comprises thorough examination, after cleansing the parts and retracting the prepuce when necessary; cutting off the long hairs about the orifice; fomentations to allay inflammation and pain; followed by astringent lotions. Tonics and demulcents should be given internally after the bowels have been cleared out by a cathartic. *Spasm and stricture of the urethra* seldom occur in the dog.

A PARASITE IN THE URETHRA caused obstruction to the passage of urine and severe urethral irritation. At length it protruded through the meatus, and its removal with the forceps gave the animal immediate relief. M. Séon, who reports the case, found the worm four inches and a half long, and considered it a strongylus; possibly it was a male *Str. gigas ?**

URETHRAL CALCULUS is generally a small cystic stone impacted in its passage. Manipulation may enable us to bring it down to the orifice of the canal and there grasp it with the forceps and so afford relief, otherwise an incision must be made on it, where it can be felt in the urethra, and removal so effected. When in the intrapelvic portion of the canal it may be detectable only on passing the catheter; there too it must be cut down upon for removal should the natural efforts not suffice to move it onwards and if it remain fixed even after the administration of chloroform and opium.

* Youatt, 'The Dog,' p. 221.

CHAPTER VIII.—THE GENERATIVE APPARATUS.

SECTION 1.—OF THE MALE.

Canis familiaris is a multiparous carnivorous mammal with zonary placenta. His generative apparatus is well developed, and in some respects, both anatomical and physiological, very remarkable. The sexual instinct runs high, and the act of copulation is prolonged. The male animal is generally allowed to remain uncastrated, and indulges in sexual intercourse freely, frequently, and with little discrimination. His genital organs occasionally suffer from excess, but probably much more frequently from enforced abstinence. The penis presents some marked peculiarities in structure,

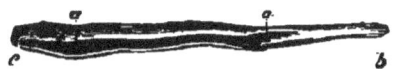

FIG. 47.—Os penis, after STRANGEWAYS.
a, groove ; *c*, base ; *b*, apex.

such as an elevator muscular arrangement for the glans and a penial bone or *penien*, through a deep groove in the lower part of which the urethra runs. This bone varies in shape in different breeds of dogs, but anteriorly terminates in a cartilaginous point, and posteriorly is directly continuous with the structure of corpus cavernosum. Lauscat describes the peculiarities of the free part of the penis of the dog in the following terms (as taken from Chauveau's Anatomy ' translated by Fleming) : " The penial bone almost entirely constitutes the base of all that portion of the penis included within the sheath; in addition this part possesses two distinct *erectile enlargements*, an anterior and a posterior. The first is analogous to that of the glans penis of the horse, and is formed by an expansion of the erectile tissue of the urethra; club-shaped at its anterior base, it has there a point suddenly bent downwards, beneath which is pierced the urethral orifice; posteriorly it is thin and partially covers the other erectile mass. The latter is supplementary; it begins at the base of the free portion of the penis, where the integument of the sheath is folded in a circular manner around it. From one to one and a half inches long; it embraces the upper border and sides of the zone; pyramidal in shape, its base, which is posterior, is three quarters to one and a quarter inches thick; in front it thins away beneath the erectile tissue of the head. Such are the two erectile masses, whose summits overlap, so that the free portion of the penis, bulging in front and still more so behind, is narrowed in the middle. Although contiguous, these two vascular dilatations are independent of each other; the posterior has, likewise, no communication with the corpus cavernosum, and possesses two particular veins, which pass backwards in a lateral groove. Each is erected separately during copulation, when they assume a large size; the great volume of the posterior enlargement prolongs the duration of this act, until flaccidity ensues. This peculiarity is a consequence of the absence of the seminal reservoirs." The familiar spectacle of a pair of dogs "locked." in coition is a consequence of the presence and physiological peculiarities of the posterior of these enlargements (Blaine attributed to the clitoris a share in producing it). When the male animal prematurely becomes moved from his natural position on the female the dilatation of the posterior part of the glans retains the penis in the vagina, and it often becomes twisted on its narrow part behind the bone, and bent backwards. This state of affairs must remain until the turgescence subsides, and any attempt to forcibly separate the animals is liable to lacerate the erectile walls of the vagino-vulval passage or to injure the penis, the parts of the bitch rather than those of the dog being liable to suffer. Throwing cold water over the animals is quite unnecessary, because if the dog be restored to its natural position separation may in a short time be effected without difficulty. Copulation is prolonged, not only to allow an ample amount of semen to gradually be expelled from the epididymis and vas deferens, but also to secure free evacuation of the secretions of the highly developed prostate.

POSTHITIS, *inflammation of the glans penis*, has already been dealt with in discussing gonorrhœa, of which it is a very frequent accompaniment. It is denoted by constant semi-erection of the penis, the glans of which is large and heightened in colour, or the seat of slight vesicular eruption around its base. There is constant irritation of the part, and not unfrequently some paraphymosis. This disease is attributed to debility, for it occurs in animals which have recently recovered from severe disease, and especially in high-bred pet dogs in which the constitution is languid and the nervous temperament predominates. The treatment is simply antiphlogistic; with subsidence of the inflammation the turgescence will pass off and œdema of the prepuce be lessened, so that the parts will resume their natural appearance.

WARTY GROWTHS of a non-malignant character are not seldom found on and within the prepuce, and sometimes on the glans. We have no evidence as to the identity of this with " sweeps' cancer " in man, although the appearances are rather similar to simple cases of the latter. The epithelial growths are confluent or separate, and occasionally form masses of a spongy character and somewhat considerable size, probably what Blaine describes as "*Polypi of the Sheath.*" These fungous growths may become ulcerated, generally in consequence of injury, and a thin watery discharge, intermingled with blood, trickles from them. Whenever, after expulsion of urine, a few drops of blood are passed, the glans penis and lining membrane of the prepuce should be examined for these growths. They should be promptly treated by removal of the larger ones with scissors or knife as required, and dressings of the smaller ones with caustic, preferably acidum aceticum. The parts should be examined daily after this, and weak solutions of nitrate of silver or zinc sulphate applied to promote healing.

CONGENITAL MALFORMATIONS OF THE PENIS are occasionally seen in dogs. Thus a case is related ('Veterinarian,' 1877, p. 249) by Gill, of Hastings, in which a pup seemed to pass his urine from the rectum in drops. Amputation of the skin over the glans penis (*circumcision*) effected a complete cure. Here there was evidently *imperforate prepuce*, of which, also, Hill relates a case.

AMPUTATION OF THE PENIS is performed on the dog in the usual manner, except that the bone must be divided with a saw or by means of a strong pair of bone forceps. Peuch and Toussaint, in describing the operation, remind us that a retraction of the urethra is apt to occur after operation and urination thereby become impeded, a contingency which must be provided against by insertion of a cannula or a short catheter, and its retention for some few days in position. In a case of cancer of the whole of the corpora cavernosa I recently removed the whole penis and testes, leaving the opening of the urethra in the perinæum. Remarkably little blood escaped on operation, but the patient being in an extremely weak state died in three hours from exhaustion.

The scrotum of the dog sometimes undergoes INFLAMMATION with very severe after-effects of a nature which has not been thoroughly explained. After a short period of severe irritation of the parts a marked erythema sets in, which runs its course rapidly and generally yields to simple antiphlogistic measures. In other cases, in consequence of neglect or constitutional peculiarity of the patient and deficiency in tone of his system, although the parts seem to be healing freely, changes are taking place which involve the deeper coats of the scrotum, extending from the inflamed skin. Thus the scrotal tissues may assume a semi-cartilaginous consistence, or their changes may seem more of a malignant character, the tissues forming a ragged ulcer, generally as a result of their having been slightly injured. This ulcer proves phagedænic, and may cause such disorganisation as rapidly to prove fatal, although it is remarked that in other cases the cancerous growth remains almost in a quiescent state until the death of the animal from other causes. What this disease is due to it is difficult to say, but it is generally attributed to derangements of the digestive organs, and, as it occurs in aged animals, to senile changes in nutrition. Treatment comprises cathartic doses to empty the bowels, followed by tonics and a liberal diet. Iodide of potassium and alkalies internally are supposed to have been administered with benefit. Locally in the second or chronic stages the application of caustics is advocated, and the diseased parts may require careful and thorough removal with the knife. This operation is generally performed together with castration, which facilitates the closure of the large resulting wound. The scrotum is sometimes affected with obstinate sores, which require great care in treatment.

CASTRATION of the dog is performed in the usual manner, preferably by scraping. In this animal, as in man, the vascular part of the cord (or simply the spermatic artery) may be ligatured, and the testis and epididymis removed at once with the knife; or the organs may be ablated by means of a small chain écraseur. But little after-treatment is required. The operation renders the animal dull and phlegmatic, inclined to sleep and grow fat, and much less companionable than previously. It should be performed only in case of the above-described disease of the scrotum, or where the testis has undergone malignant change. The testes should always be specially looked for in examining a dog as to soundness, as they are sometimes removed before sale by owners who wish to monopolise a breed. IMPOTENCE, of course, results from this last-mentioned practice, but it also is found in association with other conditions, such as excessive fatness, chronic disease of the testicles, and occasionally as an individual peculiarity, especially in over-bred animals of very valuable breeds. In cases where the testes are present occasionally good may be effected by the use of aphrodisiacs, such as cantharides, the peppers, and phosphorus pills. Generally more benefit will result from regular exercise, liberal feeding, iron tonics, and careful regulation of the bowels. Where the testes are hard and small a course of iodide of potassium may be followed by marked benefit.

The testicle is sometimes the seat of malignant disorder, *sarcocele*. Its most frequent disease is ORCHITIS, the result of blows or other injury, and also, it is said, excessive venery or sexual excitement without connection. The tense, hot, and red condition of the scrotum directs attention to the affected part, and it is easy to detect the swollen testis within it. Pressure on the gland causes acute pain. Ordinary antiphlogistic measures (especially the application of leeches) should be adopted and a cathartic administered. Sometimes suppuration of the testis occurs, and the resulting abscess, on bursting, leaves a large ragged ulcer, which heals slowly, and for which even castration may be necessary. *Cirrhosis of the testis*, a form of atrophy, is a much more frequent result.

The *spermatic cord* of the dog is very seldom the seat of disease, and scrotal and inguinal herniæ are rare in the male owing to the shortness of the bowels and the shape of the abdomen; when it does occur it is generally an epiplocele.

SECTION 2.—GENERATIVE ORGANS OF THE FEMALE.

The ovaries are situated in a special fold of the broad uterine ligaments and characterised by the shortness of this means of support. They are somewhat lobulated and produce numerous ova, several of which, passed into the horns of the uterus, may there become simultaneously impregnated. OVARIOTOMY has been advocated as a routine method of preventing the recurrence periodically of œstrum and the disabilities resulting from pregnancy; also in France it is resorted to for keeping a bitch clean and preventing rabies. It can, of course, have little, if any, value for the latter purpose. Thus it was once a practice to hunt with packs of " spayed " bitches. But it has been found that animals thus operated on are liable to disease, especially to the formation of fatty tumours; they become obese, listless, and are said not to live long. Occasionally in the present day ovariotomy has to be resorted to, as when the ovary is considered the seat of malignant disease, or when it is absolutely necessary to prevent the bitch breeding on account of injury to the pelvis or some disease of the genital passages rendering parturition impossible. The operation is performed in the way usual for small animals : The patient is placed and retained on the side ; an incision is then made antero-posteriorly in the upper part of the flank, long enough to admit the forefinger and to allow the extraction of the ovary. The finger is inserted and used as an explorer and protractor. Soon the upper ovary is felt and drawn out, a carbolised catgut ligature is placed on its ligaments, and the organ excised. The other ovary is then felt and withdrawn through the same opening, ligatured, removed, and the remaining parts returned. Sometimes the ovary is cut off without ligature, and rough operators remove the end of the uterine cornu, which is quite an unnecessary complication. The belly is usually supported with a bandage after the operation. ATROPHY of the ovaries occurs in old animals, both those which have borne young and barren bitches. Hill relates an interesting case of this nature in a Newfoundland bitch in which one ovary was merely " a hard gritty substance the size of a horse-bean embedded in a smooth round tumour of fat, the dimensions of a large walnut, and containing in the centre a cyst. The other resembled a granular fatty mass, with a full-developed ovum (*sic*, query Graafian vesicle) ready to burst on the outside " ('The Management and Diseases of the Dog'). MALIGNANT DISEASE of the ovaries also occurs, the glands are much enlarged thereby, it is diagnosable as abdominal tumour, but in less marked cases is detectable only post mortem. Ovariotomy is the only treatment likely to be attended with benefit in these cases. The Fallopian tube in the bitch is long, narrow, and wavy.

The uterus has long narrow cornua, in which the majority of the young are carried during pregnancy. It is liable to several diseases of considerable importance. METRITIS is not frequent. It is denoted by high fever and local signs of inflammation. A purulent fetid discharge *per vaginam* is generally present, and the genital passages are irritable and often simultaneously inflamed, for, except when due to accidents in parturition, this disorder depends on the injection of irritants into the vagina and uterus to bring on "heat." We have no evidence that either external injury or exposure suffices to produce inflammation of the womb except when the parts are in a state of physiological activity either from œstrum or pregnancy. When in a bitch which has recently pupped there is high fever, pain on pressure over the womb, absence of milk, and great prostration, this condition may be suspected. She should have her comforts attended to in every way, and warm cloths applied over the belly with free fomentation. The strength must be supported by tonic doses of gentian, while febrifuges also are resorted to. The bowels should be kept relaxed by means of warm enemata. Opium should be given to allay the pain, and the discharge from the uterus should be encouraged by antiseptic injections into the vagina administered warm and with the greatest care not to irritate the parts. Among the sequelæ of metritis one of the most important is ULCERATION. This generally involves only the lining mucous membrane of the womb, when there is a certain amount of fetid discharge from the parts, and the animal shows frequent œstral indications and falls away in flesh. In other cases the diseased action is much more extensive. Yeomans records the case of a small bitch in pup which about three weeks before accouchement fell four feet. Four or five days after the accident she showed a great desire to sleep, her belly became pendulous, and pressure on it caused pain, as denoted by a shrill cry. As the time of parturition approached her cries became more frequent, and she expressed much uneasiness. She brought forth four puppies, the last of which was dead, and on the following morning she had a violent fit; she was put in a warm bath and given a tablespoonful of castor-oil mixture. On the third morning she got out of her bed and ran round the place as if mad, and her eyes appeared ready to burst out of her head. The baths were repeated at intervals during the day, and in the evening she seemed better, and consciousness had returned. Next morning she was found dead, and examination of the body showed the peritoneum inflamed and a dark fluid in the abdomen, also "two large, ill-conditioned ulcers existed on one of the horns of this organ. They had completely perforated all the coats, forming a ready communication between the uterus and the abdomen" ('Vet. Record,' iii, p. 68). In ulceration of the mucous membrane cleanliness must be ensured by frequent syringing with solution of zinc chloride, and the strength of the patient supported by a course of tonics and strict hygiene.

HYDROMETRA or HYDROPS UTERI in the bitch assumes the form of accumulation of fluid in the uterine cavity, whereby distension gradually takes place, and symptoms somewhat resembling those of pregnancy may be induced; it is associated with obesity and generally also indigestion. In old bitches which have produced several litters of pups œstrum is apt to become irregular or suppressed; if this be found simultaneously with enlargement of the belly gradually increasing, and on manipulation the distension be traced to the uterus, and that organ, instead of containing several masses which feel like tumours, has an elastic resilient feel, dropsy of the womb is probably present. In its advanced stages the abdomen becomes much enlarged and markedly pendulous. The patient is prostrated and refuses food, but suffers from thirst. At length she succumbs to exhaustion, and examination shows the uterus distended with fluid of a thin watery character or thick like pus, but owing its consistency to epithelial cells as detectable under the microscope. The mucous membrane of the womb is in these cases somewhat œdematous, but no record of true œdema of the womb is to hand. The accumulation results from rigidity of the neck of the uterus with occlusion of the mouth of the organ, and so it should be dealt with by catheterism of the womb, frequently washing it out with chloride of zinc solutions, and supporting the strength of the patient by tonics.

UTERINE DISPLACEMENTS, as seen in the bitch, are of three kinds, hernia, prolapsus, and versio or twisting. HERNIA UTERI or HYSTEROCELE is common in canine practice, the displacement being generally inguinal or ventral. Rainard has recorded a case in which the uterus had been carried through the inguinal ring and was pushed backwards and appeared as a tumour at the vulva. The owner opened the swelling with a penknife, whence resulted a fistula from which a viscid fluid escaped. Rainard incised this fistula and found beneath the skin a second membrane having some analogy to it, and which afterwards proved to be the uterus ; in this was found a three or four weeks' old fœtus with its membranes, which was removed, but the bitch died the next day. Gellé describes a case of hernia of one of the uterine cornua (in which was a pup) through the mesentery. It is remarked that an essential difference exists between this lesion in multiparous animals and those which produce but one or two young at a birth. In the former the uterine cornua are long and loosely attached, and even in the unimpregnated condition of the womb they can escape through an accidental opening in the muscular walls of the abdomen or through the inguinal rings; besides, the abdominal walls are not so distant from the womb in carnivora as in herbivora. Thus, hernia occurs prior to conception or during the interval between two successive pregnancies in the bitch, and not infrequently one or more fœtuses are developed in the herniated uterine horn. Thus, a hernia, not apparently of importance, may during pregnancy increase in size as the fœtus develops in it and ultimately inconvenience be caused by it either before or at the time of parturition. Such a hernia frequently occurs in the mammary region, where its peculiar feel, and especially fluctuation on pressure at certain points, may lead to its being considered an abscess or tumour of a simple or malignant nature. The relations in development of the hernia tumour to pregnancy should suffice to ensure exact diagnosis; also, part of it may admit of being returned into the belly, and the practised hand will detect the margins of the opening through which the hernia has taken place. Corby, of Hackney, has related ('Veterinarian,' April, 1871) a case in which a herniated horn of the uterus contained a dead and decomposed fœtus, after removal of which, even, the uterine cornu could not be returned. This displacement is generally due to injuries, such as kicks and blows, but it also may result from straining in cases of constipation. In some cases the hernia is complete, even the body of the womb being contained in the sac. It is usually advisable not to interfere surgically with such a hernia. As long as the animal remains unimpregnated the tumour will cause little or no inconvenience, and even as many as three pups contained in a herniated uterus have been got rid of in the ordinary course of parturition without complication. In cases of hernia where parturition cannot take place, division of the neck of the opening may be tried and the womb returned into the belly. Metritis is rather liable to follow, and Fleming ('Veterinary Obstetrics') strongly advocates that early gastro-hysterotomy be performed in preference to herniotomy, or even that amputation of the herniated cornu be tried. Kopp recorded ('Gaz. Méd. de Strassburg,' 1875) a most interesting case of removal of three pups by the Cæsarian operation and natural birth of a fourth before the operation.

Torsio Uteri in carnivora is not the complex twisting of the whole organ on its neck, such as we see in the cow, but a contraction of the long cornua and their entanglement, either together or in the broad ligament. This lesion is rare, and hardly admits of exact diagnosis. It probably results from special activity of the vermicular contractions of the uterine cornua seen in female carnivores.

PROLAPSUS UTERI, described also as INVERSION, is not infrequent, but it is generally only a partial protrusion of the organ into the vaginal canal,* where it may interfere with urination by pressure on the meatus urinarius. Funk mentions a case in which one cornu became inverted and prevented the expulsion of the remaining fœtus from the other cornu (Fleming's 'Obstetrics'). The accident usually occurs during parturition, the result of undue straining or traction. It is most frequently seen in bitches which have had several litters of pups and which are debilitated in consequence of recent disease, or want of exercise and improper feeding. In this accident it is necessary to distinguish between protruded womb and a dropped vagina or a polypus. The latter has generally been noticed for some time, but prolapsus uteri vel vaginæ occurs suddenly at parturition. The polypus, like the vagina is smooth, soft, glistening, and feels semisolid, but, unlike the vagina, has a constricted neck and no central canal, nor can it be removed by restoration to natural position. The womb is reducible, soft, and rough ; it also generally shows the dark-coloured zone for attachment of the placenta. Thus careful examination will dispel all doubts in diagnosis. Such a lesion may be irreducible on account of swelling of the womb when it has been protruded for some time and there has been active compression on its neck. When the protruded part is of foul odour, dark colour, and much swollen, the practitioner may find it advisable to ligature round its base and amputate either directly or after the lapse of a couple of days, an operation which has been practised with complete success, as by Cross of Milan ('Youatt on the Dog,' p. 230). Generally after the womb has been thoroughly cleansed with warm water it should be restored to position by taxis ; pressure being applied at the fundus by means of a piece of wood with a padded extremity inserted through the orifice with care after being well oiled, and simultaneously the walls being worked gradually through the opening. The process of return is especially difficult and dangerous when the

* For an interesting case consult 'Veterinarian,' 1875, p. 175.

womb is much swollen and has been much lacerated by friction against the ground or otherwise; it may generally be effected by expenditure of time and the exercise of patience. The difficulty then arises of how to retain the parts when the animal strains in consequence of uterine pain or attempts to defæcate. Astringent and opiate injections into the womb will here prove useful. Mayhew has found much benefit from throwing in cold water. The patient must be kept very quiet, receive laxative diet, and the generative passages be thoroughly, though not officiously, cleansed with astringent injections of not too great strength. A small dose of castor-oil mixture will prove useful. Fecundation may occur after this serious accident, but it is advisable to keep the animal from breeding for some time, or altogether unless perpetuation of the breed be a special desideratum.

AMPUTATION OF THE UTERUS or *excision of the womb* has been performed without ill-consequences both in cases of prolapsus, and, less frequently, in conjunction with the operation of laparotomy. Numerous cases of this operation have found a place in veterinary periodical literature. Perhaps the most complicated was that recorded by Leech in vol. xxxix of the 'Veterinarian,' p. 790. The patient was a pointer bitch with irreducible uterine prolapsus. On passing the catheter the recorder found the bladder included in the protruding mass in which also, on incision through the uterine wall, was found a piece of intestine. The bladder and bowel were returned, and the hind parts of the patient raised to retain them during the performance of the operation, which was as follows: "A needle armed with a strong ligature was passed through the neck of the uterus, behind the meatus urinarius, including one fourth of its substance, which being tightly tied, the needle was again passed through another fourth and tied in the same manner; then again through another fourth in the same way, leaving one fourth up to this time free. The whole of the neck of the uterus was then included in one strong ligature, which closed the aperture into the abdomen." The organ behind the ligatures was then cut through with a scalpel and the remainder returned. The patient was well in about a fortnight. Broad prefers removal with the clamps and hot iron at a black heat as causing less suffering than the ligature and less liability to blood-poisoning. Brown relates a case ('Veterinarian,' xl, p. 845) in which there were two complications, *i. e.* fractured ilium and UTERINE TUMOUR. Growths of the latter nature are much less frequent than in the vagina. Of UTERINE INERTIA a case is related by Fleming ('Obstetrics,' p. 418) which "is interesting as showing the tendency of some animals to uterine inertia, as testifying to the great value of ergot of rye—at least, with the carnivora—its ecbolic action on animals being denied by many veterinarians; as proving that the death of one fœtus *in utero* does not always imperil the existence of the others; and as demonstrating that, contrary to what occurs in the mare and cow, fœtuses will exist in the uterus of the bitch for forty-eight hours after the expulsion of others without succumbing, even when one of their number is dead."

POST-PARTUM HÆMORRHAGE from the uterus is rare in the bitch; Mayhew has recorded a case ('Veterinarian,' xxi, p. 559). After a long assisted labour his patient was exhausted and received a stimulant, but a flow of arterial blood from the generative orifice threatened to prove serious. The patient had already shown signs of delirium, when an infusion of Tinct. Gallæ ʒss, Aquæ calidæ Oij, injected into the uterus, revived the animal by causing proper contraction of that organ.

The vagina of the bitch is long and has thick walls which are not unfrequently the seat of LACERATION. This lesion is the consequence of injury during copulation, as when the animals are dragged apart while still "locked," or it results from injuries inflicted by the passage of the fœtus or by instruments used in assisted or laboured parturition. It has been remarked by Rainard that when the vagina has been bruised or chafed during parturition in the bitch even the most trifling rupture of the walls, even though unassociated with hernia, will prove fatal, which is in marked contrast with the very considerable toleration of such injuries in the larger herbivorous mammals. We may remark, also, the great tendency there is in the bitch to the development of tumours from the wall of the vagina and vulva. Such tumours are generally described as *cancer*, but, with Mayhew, we must conclude that malignant growths are much less frequent in the genital passages of the bitch than has been supposed. In every case examined after removal, both with the microscope and by dissection, supposed epithelial cancer from this situation has turned out merely proliferation of the vulvo-vaginal walls as an immediate result of local injury; so marked is this tendency to proliferation that even after excision such tumours are liable to recur. They require in all cases to be treated in good time surgically, if left alone they increase rapidly in size, and by the acridity of their discharges produce vulvo-vaginal irritation and much inconvenience. True CANCER of the vulva and vagina may exist. It is said to result from the too free use of stimulant injections into this passage to excite the sexual desire of the animal; it probably more frequently has injuries as its immediate exciting cause.

TUMOURS IN THE VAGINA are not of rare occurrence, and they are of several kinds; *Lipomata* are more frequent in the bitch than in the female of any other known species. They vary in size and are generally removable with ease. *Condylomata* (warts) are noted by Peuch as specially liable to recur in the vagina. Sometimes small and insignificant, they in other cases may prove a serious impediment to parturition or give rise to a leucorrhœal discharge. They are irregular in outline, lobulated, and irritable. *Fibromata* also are frequently seen. True *polypus* has been recorded in many instances, and it may be classed as uterine or vaginal according to the point of attachment of its pedicle. It is smooth, vascular, and more or less resistent. Care must be taken lest it be confounded with everted bladder or prolapsed womb. These tumours when hard and well defined may be removed by operation; a true polypus may be taken off by ligature, twisting, or evulsion. The chain écraseur is the best instrument for dividing its pedicle. When the tumour is diffused, has no well-defined base, and is extensively blended with the tissues of the wall, operation (except in the case of a very small growth or of one taken early) would be too formidable an undertaking. Then the parts must be cauterised, after exposure by introduction of a speculum if necessary, and the passages kept clean by frequent washings with solutions of zinc chloride. The strength of the patient must be supported by use of tonics. LEUCORRHŒA, except when due to tumours or wounds of the vulvo-vaginal membrane, is not of frequent occurrence in bitches. When there is a discharge through the great generative opening, mainly of mucus, the parts should always be thoroughly examined and cleaned, and the cause determined. When there is simple catarrh of the membrane astringent solutions may be injected. INVERSIO v. PROLAPSUS VAGINÆ occurs in debilitated animals as a reddish or blue protuberance between the labia, varying in its degree of projection at different times and in different cases. Thus it is found especially when the animal is in "heat," and after she has several times had pups. It is not infrequently chronic in its character so that the mucous membrane becomes callous. Bull bitches are, by Mayhew, considered most liable to this displacement. Careful examination of the lesions should be made in each case to determine whether true prolapsus or vaginal tumour has to be dealt with. Treatment comprises thorough cleaning of the part (which is often injured by the animal sitting on it or dragging it on the ground), return of it to its normal position and its retention by application of astringents, such as alum solution, nitric acid with proof spirit (1-8), according to Mayhew, or ointment of tannic acid. After-treatment consists in keeping the bowels open, occasional chloride of zinc solution injections, and, especially, the administration of iron tonics. Sometimes the prolapsus occurs *post-partum*, and it may assume a chronic character, the organ protruding even beyond the lips of the vulva. When other means have failed in such a case Rainard's operation of AMPUTATION may be tried. He found that, instead of ligaturing the whole organ close to the vulva with one cord, it is better to divide the pedicle into three portions to be tied separately, so that each encloses one third of the mass. The portion of the mass beyond the ligatures may then be immediately excised. The patient is allowed to run at large, given low diet, and emollient fluids injected into the vagina. Recovery takes place very rapidly (Fleming's 'Veterinary Obstetrics'). Trusses and pessaries are not generally of value in canine practice. In France *Infibulation*, or sewing up the lips of the vulva, is advocated. The vulval opening is liable to lacerations and to tumefactions of the labia from injury or hernia. The clitoris is a flattened tubercle not often the seat of disorder. The PASSAGE OF THE CATHETER in the female is not a difficult matter; the meatus urinarius varies in depth from the external orifice from half an inch to two inches according to the size of the animal. This simple operation proves very useful in most disorders of the genital passages of the bitch; thus much inconvenience from inability to pass the urine is seen in cases of prolapsus, whether of vagina or uterus, also in cases of polypus or other vaginal tumour.

PARTURITION AND OTHER SPECIAL PHYSIOLOGICAL PHENOMENA OF THE FEMALE.—There are several matters which ought to be remembered about the physiology of the generative system of the bitch. *Œstrum* varies in the time of its occurrence and its duration in accordance with climate and surroundings, also with the general state of the health. In temperate climates it generally occurs in autumn and spring. The bitch becomes excitable and lively, her teats enlarge slightly, and then the labia and lining membrane of the vulva swell and the latter becomes red from congestion; a watery discharge from the rima appears, and it subsequently assumes a bloody character. She becomes playful with dogs, treats them most coquettishly, and will often exhibit great cunning in escaping from restraint. She is not content with a visit from one dog, but will frequently receive attentions from several of her admirers, and mix the breed in a most unsatisfactory

182   THE DISEASES OF THE DOG.

manner to any owner who desires a pure strain. The taste shown by her in selection of partners is not at all in accordance with our views; ugly curs often seem to be

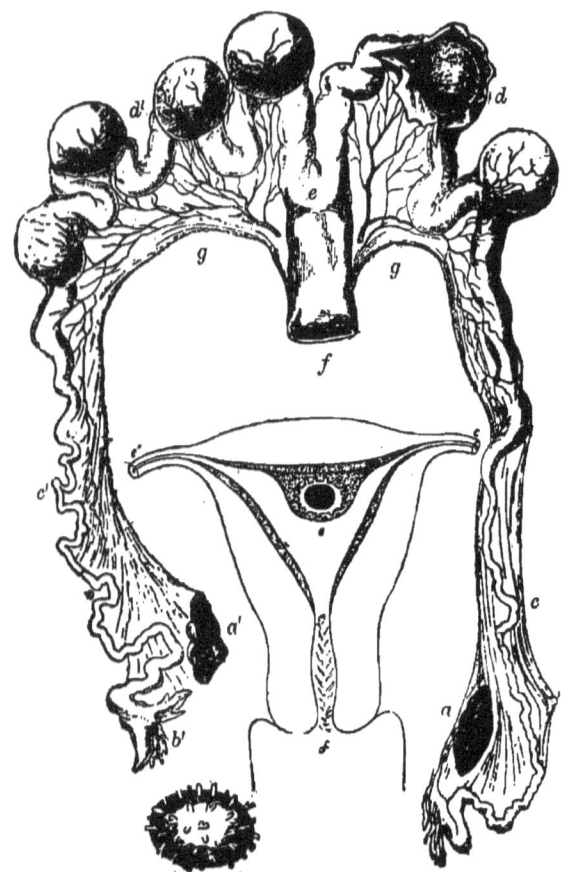

Fig. 48.—Gravid uterus of a multiparous mammal contrasted with that of the human female (from Fleming's 'Obstetrics').

$a\ a'$. Ovaries. b'. Fimbriæ. $c\ c'$. Fallopian tubes. $d\ d'$. Cornua uteri. e. Body of uterus. f. Vagina. g. Uterine broad ligaments.

most appreciated, and small bitches receive dogs so large that complications are apt to arise in parturition from the too considerable size of the progeny. As the periods of desire may extend over a week, SUPERFŒTATION is more apt to occur in canine than in other patients, and it is indicated by the throwing of pups at an interval of from two or three days to a week, the two lots sometimes differing in breed and indications of male parentage. "With the subsidence of venereal excitement in unimpregnated animals, there succeeds a period of calm, which is almost equivalent to that of gestation in impregnated creatures. And, strange to say, with bitches at the end of this interval—from the fortieth to the sixtieth day—there sometimes appear phenomena allied to the parturient period: as tumefaction of the mammary glands, followed by swelling and increase of the opening of the vulva, with reddening of the vaginal mucous membrane and the escape of a viscid fluid. The animal also acts as if about to bring forth; making a bed for her young; moving about uneasily; neglecting her food for three or four days, during which the mammæ become still more developed, firm, and elastic; the teats elongated, and the lactiferous sinuses filled with an abundance of good milk, which is easily obtained by slight pressure. If a bitch in this state is presented with a young puppy, she will take to it as if it was her own, and rear it most affectionately" (Fleming). This remarkable phenomenon is most frequently found in bitches which have been pregnant. It may necessitate care in removal of milk through the teats lest small concretions result from retention. If the bitch be not impregnated, in due course the symptoms of œstrum subside, but, it is urged, that whenever possible the animal should be allowed to breed, as sterile females are subject to degenerative changes of the ovaries and mammæ, and sometimes these parts become affected with malignant disorder. During œstrum pet bitches, especially, are liable to suffer from epileptic fits. The *absence of œstrum* at the proper periods is associated with changes, mostly of a degenerative character, of the female organs; it is not uncommonly due to dropsy of the uterus. Artificial means are sometimes adopted to excite sexual desire. These are either general or topical; the former consist in administration of stimulants, such as cubebs, cantharides, &c., the latter in the injection of irritant substances into the genital passages; sometimes the bitch is forcibly compelled to receive attentions of the male. These practices are very liable to produce local or nervous disorder, and cannot be too strongly condemned; if a bitch which it is desired should breed shows no symptoms of sexual excitement in the ordinary course of things, and no defect in her genital organs is appreciable, it is well to try the effects of a change in her system of living. Thus, an over-fed petted animal should be put gradually on less food and given regular exercise, or an excessively active hard-fed animal be put on stimulating diet and kept quiet. These measures will generally have the desired result. Some bitches are characterised by an almost *constant desire* for the male; in them there is probably some local irritation of the genitals, or there may be dropsy of the ovaries. This latter, however, is seldom present in the bitch. The bitch during œstrum and pregnancy is especially liable to mental impressions, whereby the race characters of the progeny may become vitiated. The sexual excitements of this animal are closely associated with nervous disorders.

PREGNANCY is detectable about the fourth week; the young are sometimes to be felt on abdominal exploration about this time; the belly begins to get full and round, and the teats to enlarge. The belly drops towards the seventh week and parturition occurs about the ninth week after impregnation, the range of duration of pregnancy being put by Fleming at fifty-five to seventy days. The number of young at a birth is generally seven or eight, but ranges from one up to nineteen, occasionally even more. They are some accommodated in each uterine horn, the remainder in the body of the womb. Each is developed in its own set of membranes, the placenta being a zone around the centre of the body of the young animal. The membranes and fœtus are expelled simultaneously, the pups putting in an appearance at intervals ranging from a quarter of an hour to an hour, or even longer. The immediate symptoms of parturition being imminent are enlargement of the mammæ (due to accumulation of milk), fulness of the labia, a glutinous discharge from the vagina, a desire for quietude and solitude, and for a comfortable place to litter in. *False pains* sometimes occur some time before true labour sets in, but there is then no uterine contraction appreciable simultaneous with the forcible contraction of the abdominal walls, and the os uteri has not yet relaxed. The *hygiene of pregnancy* presents no special features, but we must bear in mind the liability to nervous disorders at the time of parturition and lactation, and fortify the system against them by simple wholesome diet and full exercise. Shortly before parturition the diet should be laxative and a mild cathartic may be given two or three days before the birth is anticipated.

PARTURITION is generally accomplished by the bitch recumbent on her side. The process lasts some time in most cases and is painful, as indicated by the cries of the mother. Each expulsion is succeeded by an interval of comparative ease, during which the membranes are removed from the last expelled fœtus. Their intact condition materially facilitates birth, but is not absolutely essential. The straight and unossified condition of the pelvic symphysis materially facilitates parturition in canine patients; the offspring are numerous as a rule; each is born in an imperfect state of development, such as would be considered premature in herbivora, and consequently the skeletal structures of each are in a highly elastic and yielding condition. Hence difficulty in parturition is not very common in the bitch, and when it does occur is generally the result of exhaustion from prolonged labour pains. *Malposition of the fœtus* seldom causes trouble, the transverse presentation being the only one which gives rise to mechanical difficulties. In a small bitch which has been "lined" by a large dog (or one which is capable of begetting large progeny by the process of "throwing back") we sometimes find difficulty, and the impediment is experienced in passing over the ischium rather than at the brim of the pelvis. Fractures of the ossa innominata, with displacement or extensive deposit of callus, render parturition dangerous, and will sometimes necessitate the adoption of spaying as a measure of precaution, as has also been done with a pet bitch lined by a too-big dog. However, in the latter case the chances of the progeny not proving too big are generally good enough to render parturition worth risking. In no circumstances more than in canine obstetrics has the practitioner to remember that his duty is *to assist nature*. The case must be interfered with as little as is compatible with thorough examination, and no artificial assistance must be resorted to prematurely. The smallness of the parts in the patient both render exploration difficult and the use of instruments at once difficult and dangerous. The high nervous temperament of the bitch causes severe fever to result from any rough handling of the fœtus in its passage, or of the genital canal when thus excited. Exploration must be effected by introduction of the finger, carefully oiled, and it may be determined whether there is any mechanical impediment to the birth of the pups, whether the os uteri has properly relaxed, whether any progress has been made in delivery, and, if there is impediment, its nature may frequently be determined. Sometimes it is necessary to draw off the urine by means of a catheter, and an advantage to administer a clyster. As manipulation is liable to remove from the genital passages the viscid matter which normally lubricates them, it is necessary in most cases to apply some emollient to the passages and even to inject bland fluids into the uterine cavity. When spasm of the uterus assists to keep the fœtus in an unsatisfactory position it is advisable to resort to a bath of about 112° F. This allays irritability and relaxes the parts. At the same time it proves soothing to the bitch, but the condition of the patient while in the bath must be carefully and constantly examined lest collapse set in, and every care must be exercised to prevent a " chill " subsequent to removal. Parturition may be *premature* as a result of fright or injury, but ABORTION seldom occurs in the bitch, which is a remarkable fact when we take into consideration her high nervous organisation, and the activity of her uterine movements. Her food is not liable to contamination with ergot or other ecbolics. Also she owes this comparative immunity to her multiparity, whereby each part of the uterus acts as a semi-independent fœtal nourisher. Thus one fœtus may die and decompose without necessarily disturbing the others, and expulsion of live progeny may take place after severe operation on one of the uterine cornua. These multiple fœtuses are of small size and, as compared with those of herbivores, imperfect development. However, abortion does occur; thus Fleming relates a case in a small extremely fat bitch, which resulted at a late period of gestation from frequently ascending and descending a steep staircase.

DELAYED PARTURITION occurs in the case of a dead fœtus or when inertia uteri is present. The former state is most frequent in cases of hernia uteri, as has been already described. The latter also has been dealt with. Some discussion has taken place with regard to the value of ergot of rye as an ecbolic in canine practice. The balance of evidence tends to prove that six to eight grains of this agent administered every half hour to a medium-sized bitch in which the uterine contractions are beginning to fail, proves most useful. Of course it is not admissible in cases of mechanical impediment, and should be resorted to only under professional supervision. The flagging powers of the bitch may be supported by brandy and beef-tea, frequently administered, in doses ranging from a dessertspoonful to a teaspoonful.

OPERATIVE INTERFERENCE seldom is required. *Embryotomy* is difficult and seldom needed, for when the fœtus is within reach it can usually be extracted by mild traction after adjustment. Those fœtuses which lie in the depths of the horns of the womb are far out of reach until moved from their position into the body of the organ, and even there they are barely accessible; when the young animal becomes impeded in its passage through the vagina, the forceps, crochet, and other implements may be resorted to. If the head is too large and incompressible, as it is apt to be in the bull and pug breeds, *Cephalotomy* may be tried and the excessive size of the skull reduced after evacuation of its contents by puncture or incision. Many positions of the fœtus which need adjustment in the larger animals are manageable by direct traction in the carnivore. This traction must be gentle and only at the time of the throes; the limbs may sometimes be secured by a loop of worsted, but Mayhew's parturition instrument is preferable. He urges that the worsted skein sometimes cuts through the limb to which it is fastened, and when introduced into the vagina it soon becomes moist, adheres to the finger and cannot be detached from it; whereas pliable wire does not become moist and is readily adjustable.

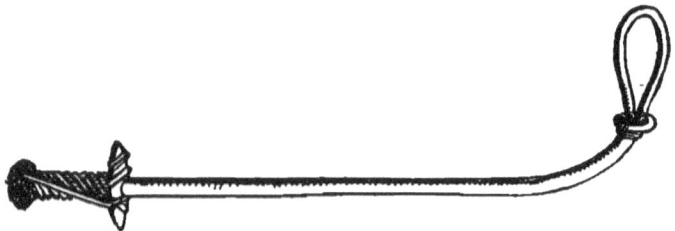

FIG. 49.—Parturition Instrument (MAYHEW).

The instrument consists of a tube of polished metal which is at one end curved to suit the line of the pelvis, and at the other is grooved and has a small cross-bar. Into the tube a piece of zinc wire is introduced, so as to double and form a loop at the bent extremity, the ends of the wire coming forth at the other. One of the ends of the wire is twisted into the groove so as to render it fast; and that being done the instrument may when required be introduced with the loop of wire upon the point of the finger, and, the paw it is to be desired to fix being felt, the finger is withdrawn and the instrument moved forward. The free end of the wire is then pulled to render the hold firm, after which it is twisted round the projecting bar and made secure. The tube assists us in guiding the loop, which, being once fixed, can be made secure, and so traction does not afterwards further tighten it (Mayhew,

'Dogs'). Fleming draws attention to the fact that in small bitches the use of forceps increases the difficulties of parturition, and that therefore extractors are, in such diminutive animals, much preferable. The *extractors* are to be fixed on the neck of the foetus with a view to the exercise of direct traction. Two kinds are mentioned, the complex one of Defays, and the very simple one of Breulet (which closely resembles Mayhew's instrument). Of *forceps*, as available for larger bitches, there are several kinds, those like polypus forceps, such as Hill's and Defays', and that modified from one in use in human practice by Weber. Defays points out that it is most difficult to apply an instrument in shape like that of the accoucheur's ordinary forceps, owing to the neck of the foetus in carnivora being so thick, and the difference in volume between it and head far less than in the human foetus. So that when the forceps is used, the bow of the blades presses on the neck, slips under the throat, and the head escapes from them (Fleming, 'Obstetrics'). When the pup is dead, delivery is more difficult than when living; rupture of the membrane generally occurs with those which come last when several are produced at a time, but ruptured membranes are almost invariably found when the pup is dead. The gradual passage of a decomposed foetus is much rarer in the bitch than in the cow, but it occurs when the young one has been contained in a hernia. The crochet, as used in extraction by Mayhew, is described in the 'Veterinarian' for 1847. It is a human crochet

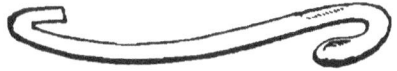

FIG. 50.—Crochet (MAYHEW).

altered to order. "A piece of stout steel wire, about twelve inches long, flattened at one extremity. Both ends are crooked and made perfectly smooth or blunt, the flattened hook being the larger of the two . . . As the pup, in consequence of the weakness of the abdominal

190   THE DISEASES OF THE DOG.

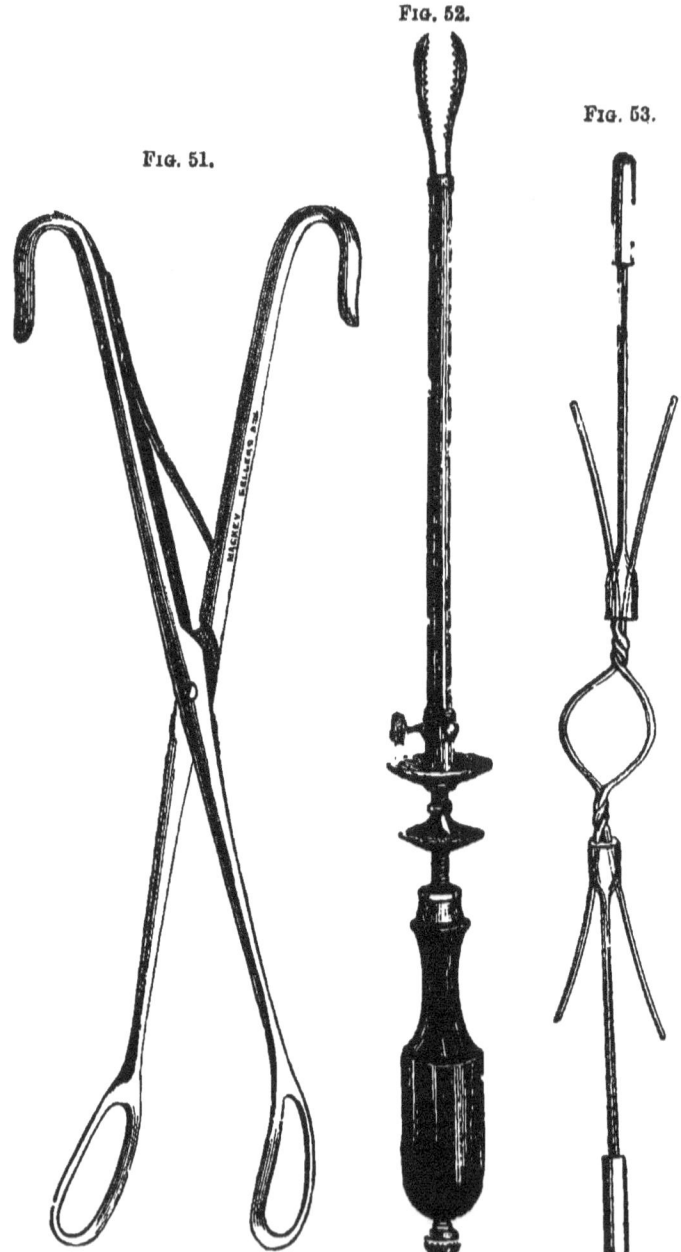

FIGS. 51—53.—Forceps and Extractors (FLEMING).

THE GENERATIVE APPARATUS. 191

Fig. 54.

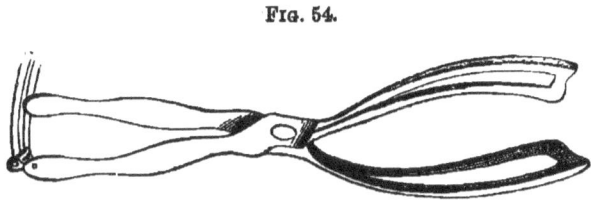

Fig. 55.

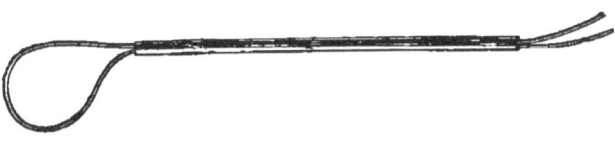

Fig. 56.

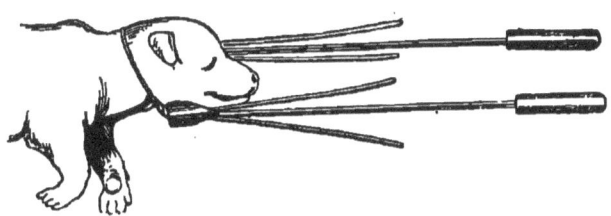

FIGS. 54—56.—Forceps and Extractors (FLEMING).

parietes in the bitch, often is felt lying below the level of the symphysis, a dip or lateral bend is given to the hooks. So simple is the crochet, which ought to be highly polished in order to secure its being perfectly smooth. It is first warmed and greased, then introduced with the index finger of one hand, while the other guides the instrument into the womb. The fœtus is to be first felt, and this is the more readily done if an assistant supports and compresses the abdomen. When the finger has ascertained that the pup is favorably placed, the hook (and I generally use the flattened extremity of the instrument) is to be pushed forward and then retracted, until the operator is aware that a firm hold has been obtained.

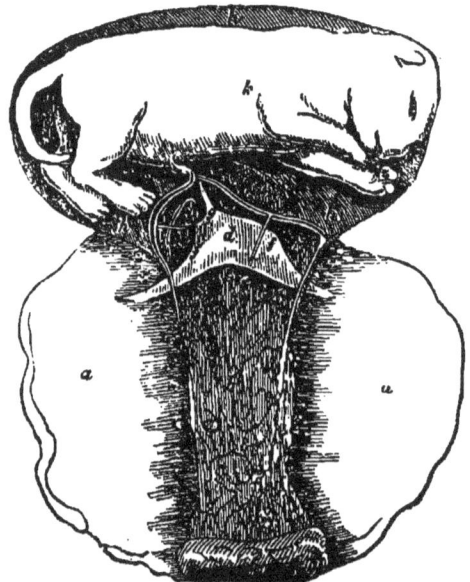

FIG. 57.—Fœtus in its membranes (FLEMING).
a. Chorion. k. Fœtal pup. h. Amnion. d. Umbilical vesicle.
g. Umbilical cord. b. Zonary placenta.

The purchase being secure, the finger is to be employed to prevent the fœtus from escaping, by pushing it against or towards the point of the crochet and holding it there. Traction is now made steadily and in the proper direction ; and the assistant at the same time, by manipulating the belly, facilitates the delivery of the bitch, which should be in a standing position, not upon its back."

The newly-born pup is from six to eight inches in length, and its placental zone is remarkable for a green colour due to chlorophyll. The principal other respect in which the membranous appendages of the young differ from those of the foal or calf is in the persistence of the umbilical vesicle until birth with its considerable omphalo-mesenteric vessels. This is another result of short gestation, also it has been found that the bitch gives less nutriment in proportion to her weight to the fœtus *in utero* than any other of our domesticated animals.

MONSTROUS CONDITIONS of pups, although by no means rare, are not often the cause of difficult parturition. The irregularity in development and form generally appears as excess in number of digits, deficiencies of digits or limbs, absence of face, and other minor additions to, or defects of, parts. The comparative infrequence of double fœtuses may depend on the several in a multiparous animal occupying their respective divisions of the uterine cavity, whereas in animals ordinarily uniparous twin progeny lie together in the cavity of the womb. This explanation, of course, would not suffice in the case of a double ovum. It will be enough if we here notice two irregularities with regard to the development and position of the fœtus. *Moles* or *anidian monsters* have been found by Rainard in the uterus of the bitch, most frequently in the last dilatation of one of the horns, rarely in both, " and sometimes between two dilatations which contain living fœtuses. They are spheroidal, soft, irregular in shape, and look like flesh ; they appear to be composed of fibres running in every direction. In the dilatation of the horn containing them, traces of a zonular uterine placenta have been observed." They were considered embryos of checked or perverted development. EXTRA-UTERINE FŒTATION.—A case is on record in which a fœtus, of which the skeleton only seemed to remain, was found in the mesentery of a small bitch, thirteen years old; it could hardly have been a *fœtus in fœtû*. Carter, of Burnley, describes ('Veterinarian,' 1885, p. 403) a case of tubal fœtation in a mastiff bitch. For six months or more since pupping, she had an offensive greenish-yellow discharge through the vagina; she died suddenly. Post-mortem examination showed the uterus much distended with pus, its lining membrane flabby, pale, and thickened, and with numerous, short, fawn-coloured hairs firmly embedded in its substance. The left Fallopian tube very much elongated and distended in its centre, resembling a horse's stomach in shape, containing pus and six bones (humerus, sacrum, and four cranial), completely ossified and partially covered with fawn-coloured hair. The lining membrane of the tube was thickened, corrugated, and deeply grooved; probably earlier in this case an "abdominal tumour," supposed to be uterine, might have been diagnosed and the CÆSAREAN OPERATION performed. This most formidable effort of surgery has been frequently attempted in emergency on the bitch, generally without success, because only after the vital powers have begun to flag. The fatality to the mother is put at 60 per cent. by Franck, who considers that this might be lessened if the operation were performed on the right side, and with antiseptic precautions. He quotes four cases out of forty-eight in all, in which the female and one or more of the young were preserved alive; of these four patients three were bitches. Feser has recorded* a case in which three puppies were extracted through an incision made in the left flank; a live one from each cornu, and a dead one, with its head turned back, from the body of the womb. The uterus and Fallopian tubes were removed with the écraseur, the arteries ligatured, the abdominal wound sutured, and ice applied. In sixteen days the bitch had quite recovered, and the pups were reared artificially. The same operator saved four puppies and the bitch in another case similarly treated. Adam†

* 'Thierärztliche Mittheilungen der Münchenerschule,' H. iii, pp. 296 and 298.
† 'Briefliche Mittheilung.'

successfully operated from the *linea alba* behind the umbilicus. The bitch again became pregnant, but died in pupping. The indications for "gastro-hysterotomy" are : —that delivery *per vias naturales* be impracticable, either through mechanical impediment or on account of the fœtal mass being too large or impacted, that the patient be not too exhausted to rally (even then it may be performed to save the puppies), that the animal has no chance of safe natural delivery. The operation is a laparotomy performed in the usual manner, and the incision into the uterus should be closed with catgut sutures, or, when considered necessary, the whole organ should be removed. Cases of uterine hernia are those in which this operation is most frequently performed with benefit on the bitch.

The AFTER-TREATMENT OF PARTURIENT ANIMALS is simple in the extreme; it consists in avoidance of deleterious influences, in good feeding, dry housing, and not too great a strain on the milking powers. When there is a large family of pups, a foster-mother may be required for some of them, for a bitch required to bring up too many whelps will suffer from the constitutional strain in supplying enough milk and will be liable to epilepsy. It should be remembered that the milk of the foster-mother may convey disease, and even, it is considered, constitutional peculiarities, to the suckler. When a bitch will not take to a foster-pup she may generally be persuaded to do so by removal of her own and by sprinkling the youngster with some of her milk. The bitch often devours the fœtal membranes, and, by a strange perversion of natural instinct, may kill and eat her own progeny. This very unsatisfactory tendency is much more marked in some females than in others, and has been attributed to indigestion and thirst. Such an animal should receive a cathartic or emetic dose and be carefully watched; the desire to do mischief to the young will soon pass off. She should be kept quiet.

There is for some days after parturition a discharge from the vagina, the lochia corresponding to those of the human female; the modified portions of the uterine membrane, *decidua vera,* which lay against the placentæ, are shed, and the womb gradually resumes its ordinary non-pregnant characters.

APPENDIX.—ORGANS AND PROCESS OF LACTATION AND
THEIR DISORDERS.

The mammary glands are eight to ten in number, arranged in double series along the under surface of the trunk, four being pectoral, four abdominal, and two inguinal. They are simple as compared with the elaborate corresponding organs in the cow, but, nevertheless, each is a small complete gland and has a teat with orifices numbering from eight to ten. The milk produced by these organs is specially rich, containing a very considerably larger proportion of solids than that of almost any other domesticated animal, the preponderance being in casein and fatty matters. Fleming alludes to an idea prevalent in a part of France where women suckle puppies, that the latter suffer from rickets when thus weaned. The use of pups by women to remove surplus milk from their mammæ is also adopted in Burma, where small fancy dogs are much appreciated for the purpose.

RETENTION OF MILK is apt to occur when non-parturient animals commence to have activity of the mammary glands, or in those mammæ which are least appreciated by the pups (generally the pectorals). Such retained milk is very apt to form small hard concretions in the teats which obstruct the flow of any milk subsequently formed, and so may give rise to so-called "milk abscess." To avoid this the teats should be regularly examined, and any excess of secretion removed by pressure from above downwards. The state of these parts should be constantly looked to in every bitch suckling pups, or in which any signs of spurious pregnancy have been manifested. If these concretions actually have formed, the best treatment is prompt surgical removal, which, although it seems somewhat heroic in principle, will be found the best plan in the long run. If they be very soft and evidently recent, good may result from alkaline injections into the milk-ducts, but this is a difficult and tedious process and good very seldom results from it. Mammitis may be produced by these accumulations when they are left unattended to, and very serious tumours of the gland may follow. MAMMITIS results from injuries and from exposure during lactation, in addition to the above-mentioned cause. It gives rise to serious and extensive changes in the affected gland, which changes are often described as scirrhous cancer, and the parts removed accordingly. Inflammation of one of these glands is readily detectable by high fever and the local signs of inflammation. The milk from the affected gland or glands will sometimes be found bloody and is generally mixed with pus. The results of the disorder are obstinate *lacteal fistulæ*, openings of the sinuses at the base of the teats (through which milk constantly drains and proves an impediment to healing) or abscess, or induration with functional obliteration of the gland. Ordinary antiphlogistic treatment having been carefully and diligently resorted to in the acute stages, further measures must be adapted to the progress of the case. Abscesses must be freely opened; scirrhous parts must be dressed with tincture of iodine or with iodide of potassium ointment. Fortunately, obliteration of one of the mammæ is not so serious a matter in the bitch as is " loss of a quarter " in a cow. MALIGNANT GROWTHS are frequent in the mammæ of the bitch, although probably less so than is generally supposed, as ordinary indurations of the glands are taken for them. It is certain that a simple inflammation of one of the glands may determine the development of malignant growth in it. The same result is apt to follow injury, as by the pups in suckling, blows, kicks, and other violence. Malignancy is determined by the rapid growth of the injured part and by its undergoing ulceration as a result of even slight contusions or wounds after inflammation has been controlled; surgical removal is the only treatment to be relied on in such cases. The excision of a cancerous gland is conducted on general surgical principles; the operation is severe. It should be performed under chloroform, and all hæmorrhage zealously controlled by styptics. Unless all the cancerous growth be removed at once it is very apt to grow again rapidly. TUMOURS IN THE MAMMARY GLAND vary much in their characters; perhaps the most remarkable change which they undergo is into spiculæ of bone.* This is not uncommon. The system of the patient operated on for these tumours will generally require support by good food and a course of tonics. We can "dry up" a bitch by removing the pups and giving a cathartic, and milking daily. The teats are sometimes the seat of WARTY GROWTHS and obstinate CRACKS, but these lesions are rare in the bitch, and resemble those seen in other species and need the same treatment.

* Ainslie recorded an interesting case in the 'Veterinary Record' for 1847, p. 206.

CHAPTER IX.—THE NERVOUS SYSTEM.

ALL the evidence available tends to show that the dog, more than any other of our domesticated animals, is liable to disorder of the nervous system, especially of the central masses of the cerebro-spinal portion. The brain is specially well developed in the species Canis, much more so, too, in some breeds than in others.* Thus the ladies' toy terrier, the pug, the Italian greyhound, and other fancy strains, have larger brains in proportion to their bodies than have dogs of the chase. In some this cerebral development is all but abnormal, and is associated with high nervous temperament, which must be taken into consideration both in manipulation and treatment of the animal. There can be no doubt that such dogs sometimes feign to be ill, that they sometimes make simple cases seem very urgent by their demeanour, that they require to be dealt with firmly but gently, and not allowed to take advantage; moreover, we must regulate any doses and medicines used by careful consideration of the special temperament of the patient. A harsh word may throw a dog into convulsions, and rough, hasty approach of the canine surgeon will often bring about a most intense state of nervous excitement. *Neuralgia*, even, has been described in the bitch. Fleming records the case of an Irish setter in which fits of howling and screaming indicative of pain used to come on suddenly, and the head was bent to one side when she moved. She gradually rose up on her hind legs, fell backwards, and lay howling for a considerable time. No cause could be

* Master MacGrath, the celebrated Irish greyhound, had a very large brain for a dog of his breed, but not exceptional for the species. Arloing has utilised the conclusions arrived at by physiologists as to cerebral localisation successfully for exact diagnosis of cerebral lesions in dogs.

found sufficient to account for these peculiar symptoms, but a cathartic dose and a blister along the side of the face, followed by carbolic applications, effected a perfect cure.* Williams alludes, in his 'Veterinary Medicine,' to there being certainly some instances of what might be considered aberrations of intellect or morbid fancies, especially in the dog, whereby the docile become ferocious, the good-tempered irritable, and the intelligent stupid, and notwithstanding the varieties in temperament and intelligence of animals the purely mental diseases are absent. There can be no doubt, considering the high mental qualities shown by some dogs and the zeal with which they participate in our sports and labours, that the study of nervous disorders in them is at present in a very elementary state. There are certain conditions which are symptoms of disease rather than independent pathological states which must be now dealt with. EPILEPSY is of frequent occurrence, and it is commonly spoken of as "fits." It is a loss of consciousness associated with convulsions dependent on irritation either directly of the central nervous organs or peripheral. Thus it is seen in young animals from teething or worms, and sometimes occurs in the bitch from parturition. A depraved state of the blood, as in distemper, may cause it, and not unfrequently it results from anæmic or plethoric states. When a bitch is overmilked by too many pups being kept on her, or by want of proper nutrition, she is apt to have fits which may prove fatal. Blows on the head induce changes of the brain-substance and membranes indicated by epilepsy, and it is seen to follow unusual exertion or excitement, especially in animals "out of condition." Thus, sporting dogs suffer from epilepsy at the commencement of the season, and it is found in carriage dogs, especially when the weather is hot. Constipation is a predisposing cause, and Dr. Brown-Séquard has proved that it may depend on lesions of the spinal cord. *Symptoms.*—The fits most frequently come on when the animal has been exerting itself. Its pace becomes slow and it looks distressed, although it appa-

* Hill's 'Dog.'

rently was in perfect health at starting. It soon falls, and its limbs are rigid and quivering or violently convulsed, it foams at the mouth, champs the jaws, and may bite its tongue severely; its eyes protrude, or the lids are closed and the eyeballs rolling spasmodically, or some strabismus is present. Urine and fæces are expelled involuntarily, and, rarely, sweats moisten the body. The pulse is irregular in the extreme, very fast, and sometimes imperceptible; the respiration is stertorous. The fit may pass off in a very short time, five minutes to a quarter of an hour, and the animal seem dazed and inclined to run away, or very weak and anxious to sleep. In other cases there is a succession of fits, which may prove fatal. *Diagnosis.—* These fits are erroneously considered rabies, and many dogs have been destroyed for them accordingly. The popular idea of "mad dogs" foaming at the mouth and falling in fits, also biting anyone touching them during convulsions, and running away, is exactly realised by the phenomena in epilepsy, but, as we have previously seen, the rabid dog does not generally show its disease in this way. A distinction is sometimes drawn between attacks of epilepsy as above described and those of VERTIGO, in which there are no convulsions but simple syncope, a temporary loss of consciousness, or fainting fit lasting a few minutes and leaving the animal apparently as well as ever, though a little dazed. Vertigo is attributed by Williams to disease of the heart or pericardium, by Hill to tight collars, bronchocele, and stomach disorder. To these must be added liver derangement (especially softening), one of the principal causes of the giddiness in the tropics. Mégnin has described an epileptiform disease of dogs which proved to be auricular acariasis and must not be mistaken for true epilepsy. *Treatment.*—In slight cases of epilepsy, and in vertigo, such simple measures as cold water applications to the head and quietude, also loosening the collar will suffice, but invariably some change should be made in the management of the animal. Mayhew, in his usual curious style, draws attention to some of the rough-and-ready suggestions which are likely to be made to the owner of a dog which becomes affected with a fit in the public thoroughfares; such are to lance the mouth, slit the ear, cut a piece of the tail off, give a full dose of salt and water or a lump of tobacco, or throw the patient into an adjacent pond, or rub his nose with syrup of buckthorn. It will be observed that some of these measures are directed to the removal of blood, which is seldom necessary. Mayhew's suggestion that in hot weather owners walking with dogs in the country should always carry about with them laudanum, ether, and an injection syringe to administer a dose with, will hardly be adopted, although he, "armed with this, fearlessly faced the disorder which other veterinary surgeons dread." The animal should, when seized with a fit, be secured to prevent his running away when it is over, cold water should be thrown on his head, and protection from the sun afforded. He should then be taken home or to an infirmary quietly, and a dose of cathartic medicine given. Strict attention to hygienic measures, and the removal of all operative causes of this disorder, will be of benefit, and belladonna or chloral may be resorted to in cases when the fits tend to be successive. In chronic tendency to fits the effects of a seton or a blister to the

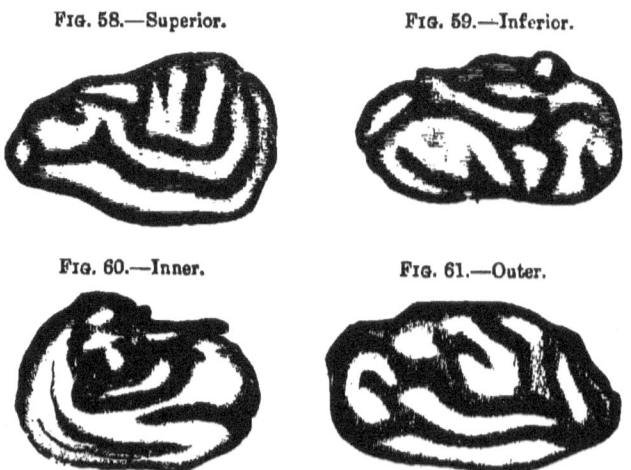

Figs 58—61.—Aspects of cerebral hemispheres of cat (life size).

FIG. 62.—Superior.

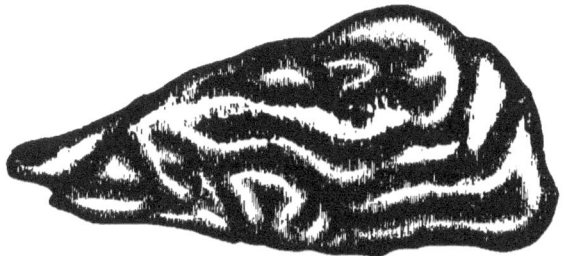

FIG. 63.—Inferior.

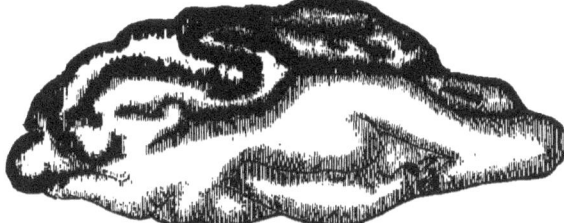

FIG. 64.—Inner.

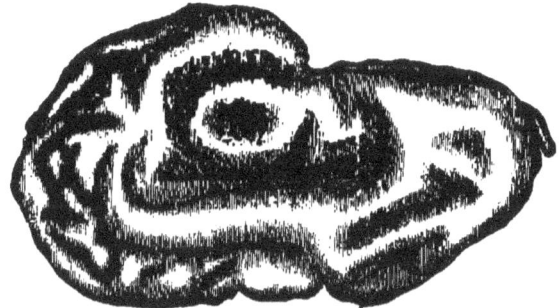

FIG. 65.—Outer.

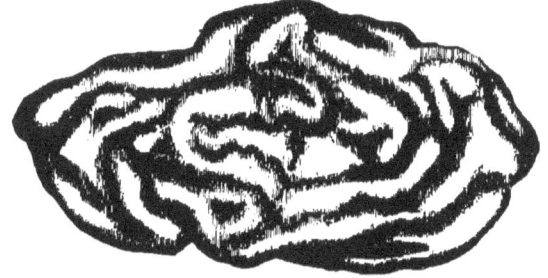

FIGS. 62—65.—Aspects of cerebral hemispheres of dog (life size).

head should be tried and the patient put through a course of nitrate of silver in quarter-grain doses, or of sulphate of iron or bromide of potassium.

APOPLEXY, the extravasation of blood on or in the brain, is occasionally seen in the dog as an after-effect of parturition. In short-necked dogs, too, it results from tight collars or the animal straining at his chain in hot weather, it may supervene on severe exertion during summer, and it is seen in many cases of sunstroke, especially those which last for a long period; plethora and insufficient exercise for some time predispose to it, and it especially occurs in dogs which are fat and somewhat old, probably a consequence of degenerative changes in the walls of their cerebral blood-vessels either from senility or adiposity. It is said to follow severe straining in obstinate constipation and also in parturition. In the latter case it is also attributable to other causes. Thus sudden suppression of milk in an animal at about the time it is giving birth to pups, premature deprivation of the young, and a plethoric state of the body before lying in, are the special causes operative in this case. In typical cerebral apoplexy, the pulse is slow and full, but we very seldom get uncomplicated cases of this disorder; thus, with the sudden and complete loss of consciousness which results when the cerebral vessels give way, there may be found a quick small pulse. The breathing is usually stertorous and the pupil dilated, the visible mucous membrane congested, and urine and fæces passed involuntarily. These symptoms may be complicated with those of coma or with a certain amount of delirium. Treatment consists in the prompt administration of the pure stimulants, such as ammonia, the narcotics being avoided, since they tend to increase the cerebral congestion. Cold water should be applied to the head directly the animal becomes unconscious, and this is a case in which general bleeding is likely to be attended with benefit. Later, a blister to the upper part of the head may effect some good result, but the patient generally dies before it has time to act. In the parturient form death is less rapid, and, indeed, the symptoms are very complicated. The main resource in such cases should be stimulants in small doses frequently repeated, a full cathartic, and careful removal of any milk formed in the mammæ. It seems to be generally accepted that this *parturient apoplexy* is the same as the disease of that name which affects the cow; but that is a point which certainly has not been proved, indeed it is doubtful whether any true apoplectic lesions take place in the majority of cases, the disease seems more a puerperal fever.

INJURIES TO THE HEAD induce cerebral symptoms varying with the amount of the lesions and their distribution. In addition to the more superficial effects, the following may be noted : concussion of the brain, compression, lesions of the meninges, and apoplexy. The animal in either case is usually prostrated by the blow, and it requires great care to determine the exact degree of injury in the dog. It is generally considered that the stunned condition, loss of motor and sensory power, which results immediately on the injury, is due to concussion, that insensibility and apoplectic symptoms occurring a short time after the injury, are the result of extravasations, and that they are also found in compression due to a depressed portion of bone in fracture. As in true apoplexy, the compressed part of the brain may in time accommodate itself to the pressure on its surface, and recovery take place, but often with the unequal power of the two sides of the body indicated by the animal involuntarily inclining towards the side where the compression has occurred. In a case described by Professor Simonds, the skull of which is in the museum of the London College, there was permanent derangement of the locomotory powers after fracture of the skull of a toy terrier by a quoit parallel with and to one side of the sagittal suture, and the successful removal of the depressed fragment. The animal when called used to wag its tail and run in the opposite direction. In cases of concussion, the loss of consciousness gradually wears off, and there is a tendency to the development of indications of inflammatory disorder of the encephalon. In such an emergency the animal should be kept very quiet, and his head bathed constantly with cold water, leeches may be applied to it, and in cases taken early, even small doses of Liq. Ammoniæ given. The injury should receive the most careful attention, it should be fully explored with a view to the detection of fracture and removal of the depressed portions with the elevator and trephine, *sec. art.* It should then be treated antiseptically and so as to control any tendency to inflammation. The supervention of ENCEPHALITIS will be indicated by excitement, and convulsions, followed at a short interval by coma and paralysis, according as the meninges and the brain-substance are gradually involved. An interesting case of injury to the brain and its membranes is recorded in the 'Veterinarian,' 1843, from M. Leblanc. Although given *in extenso* by Youatt and Hill it will bear summary here. Autopsy showed that the meninges of the *left* cerebral lobe were not thicker than one membrane usually is, and the corresponding brain-substance seemed firmer than normal. The cerebral fissures and vessels of the left lobe were small. The patient was three years old and subject to epilepsy. His final fit was followed by a loss of the usual lively appearance of the eye, and the eyelids being often closed and the animal spiritless, drowsy, and subject to clonic spasms of the muscles of the head and chest. He always lay on his left side, and in walking he exhibited a marked propensity to turn to the left. He latterly gyrated to the left and kept walking until worn out. He continued his course regardless of obstacles, and at last he seemed to simply turn as on a pivot to the left. He became very thin. Messrs. Gowing ('Veterinarian,' 1870) relate a case of effusion of pus into the left arachnoid sac, probably the result of injury. The dura mater was diseased and there was a recent hæmorrhagic clot in the left corpus striatum. The patient had lost his sight, both pupils being dilated; he advanced cautiously, inclining neither to right nor left, and was obedient to his master's call. He slightly recovered use of the left eye. He fell somewhat suddenly on the left side after this improvement, and the muscles of his neck became rigid, and his nose pointing upwards.

He soon afterwards died. In encephalitis but little can be done beyond cold applications to the head, enemata and laxatives, and the administration of aconite or prussic acid in small doses frequently repeated. In chronic cases, such as the two above referred to, counter-irritation by setons, blisters, &c., may be resorted to, and the bromide of potassium given internally.

HYDROCEPHALUS, dropsy of the meninges or of the ventricles of the brain, seems to be invariably congenital, and especially found in high-bred artificial varieties, such as French poodles and toy terriers. In a case given in detail in the 'Veterinary Record,' vol. iii, the animal was three months old; he lay on his side and made frequent ineffectual attempts to rise; in doing so he struck his head against the ground. Placed on his feet he ran with his head down, crossing his legs, reeling to and fro, and at last fell. His appetite was ravenous, and on anything being put in his mouth he would grind his teeth most painfully. His special senses were unaffected. If he attempted to look up his eyes rolled upwards. He was destroyed, as all such patients should be. Somnolence, lethargic movements, and a want of vigour are found in these cases, and generally paralysis precedes their early death.

PARASITES have been found in the cranium of the dog, but they are rare. They give rise to the symptoms of increasing compression, such as inclination to walk in a circle, gradual loss of sight, dulness, and want of vigour. The parasite is the gid hydatid (*Coenurus cerebralis*), that which is found so often in the sheep.

The spinal cord of the dog is disordered in very many cases, and in certain blood diseases, such as rabies, distemper, and rheumatism, it is specially liable to derangement. PARALYSIS, either general or local, is in the dog more frequently a sequela or concomitant of these diseases than due to other causes, and it generally when local assumes the form of paraplegia, although hemiplegia also is seen more frequently than in the horse or ox. Not only is paralysis from direct derangement of the cord found in the dog, but also the excentric or reflex form. Thus teething, irritation from worms in the alimentary canal, and pregnancy, also accumulation of hard irritant fæces in the large intestine, may cause more or less complete paralysis. The frequency of paralysis in connection with inflammatory or other painful disorders in the bowels in the dog is a point of interest and importance. Acute palsy in him is very frequently accompanied by vomition and intestinal pains. Amaurosis may be present in paralysed animals; both motion and sensation or either of them may be lost either completely or partially. As almost every form of debility in the dog culminates in the loss of motor power, especially of the hind limbs, so the anæmia of extreme obesity will be found a fruitful source of paralysis. Treatment consists in determining the cause of the loss of power and its removal. The cause may be depressed fracture, injury to nerves or spinal cord, derangement of the alimentary canal, and so on. When the special cause of the case has been removed or palliated, a cathartic may be given with a view to the expulsion of any possible source of irritation from the bowels. The animal must receive simple but nutrient food, be kept warm and treated with tonics. When the loss of power is persistent or recurrent, counter-irritation must be applied over the part supposed to be injured or the main seat of disease. Blisters or setons thus prove useful. In confirmed cases electric shocks have been resorted to with benefit, and strychnia in half-grain doses has assisted to restore the animal to health. In acute cases, where much irritation of the cord and its membranes has to be dealt with, hydrocyanic acid doses may be tried. We must always remember that in the dog paralysis is very liable to recur, and that, therefore, a course of iodide of potassium (internally and externally) is likely to be of benefit to promote absorption of deposits. During the progress of these cases the liability of the patient to bedsores must be constantly kept in mind; he should be frequently turned over from the side on which he is recumbent. The urine may be drawn off with a catheter frequently. Youatt relates an interesting case in which skin disease and paralysis alternated with one another. Blaine speaks of the operation of *acupuncturation* for long-continued rheumatic weakness of the loins and hind extremities. In one case "a needle was introduced nearly half an inch into the muscular masses in three separate parts of the back opposite the psoæ muscles with but trifling amendment, but the introduction of it into the inner and outer surfaces of the thighs, rather more than half an inch, was more beneficial." Laxatives, light diet, and careful exercise are very conducive to recovery when the loss of power is but partial.* In the 'Veterinarian' for 1878, at p. 780, are recorded M. Mauri's views on LOCOMOTOR ATAXY in the dog. He is a careful and experienced observer, worthy of close attention. He has described as PUERPERAL ECLAMPSIA a disorder of the nervous system, of which he has recorded a number of instances, as quoted in Fleming's 'Veterinary Obstetrics.' The patient generally became affected some twelve or fifteen days after pupping, and the symptoms supervened suddenly. They were anxiety, panting, tongue pendent, and frothy saliva flowing from the mouth, consciousness, mucous membranes congested; sometimes plaintive cries and restlessness. Urine suppressed; bowels constipated. These general signs were associated with clonic spasms of the limbs, or paraplegia, or a certain amount of want of control over the movements of the limbs, and sometimes the eyes roll in the sockets. These symptoms disappeared almost as rapidly as they set in, generally as a result of narcotic doses and sinapisms along the spine. Recovery is sometimes preceded by profound coma. In a case recorded by Lafitte, supposed to be of this disease, the two pups suckling the patient suffered, one, a female, died after three attacks on successive days, the other, a male, had two attacks.

CHOREA (or *St. Vitus's dance*) is a general affection of the nervous system which is found in especial relations

* Stross, of the Vienna School, has placed on record a case of spinal pachymeningitis in the dog.

with a debilitated state of the constitution in general. Thus it most frequently follows the depraved and impoverished condition of the blood seen in distemper, although it is said also to immediately follow injury involving the cerebro-spinal central masses. It may be general or local, and the latter usually terminates in the former. One limb only may be affected or both fore or both hind. In yet other instances the muscles of the face only are involved. The derangement consists in clonic spasms which may persist even during sleep. The general disorder is described as a paralysis agitans and usually proves fatal, but the more local varieties of the disease are often amenable to treatment. The effect produced on the appearance and actions of the animal by the clonic spasms is characteristic; the patient is often highly irritable, and he cries plaintively in his sleep. In other cases he seems in excellent spirits and has a very good appetite; the constant motion wears him out and he succumbs to exhaustion, preceded in most cases by paralysis. Dr. Gowers and Mr. Sankey have examined the pathological anatomy in canine chorea and reported their results before the Royal Med. and Chir. Society of London (*vide* ' Veterinary Journal,' vol. v). They examined two cases. In one the movements were confined to one foreleg. In it the medulla oblongata was normal, and the other centres were but slightly affected. On examination of the spinal cord it was found that the large cells of the cervical region were very granular and appeared swollen, more so on the right side than on the left; there was a slight increase in the minute nuclei of the anterior (inferior) right column; in the anterior lumbar region the nerve-cells of the right superior vesicular column were more granular than those of the left. The second case was a sequela of distemper. The twitchings were general, the limbs, especially the hind ones, were very weak and the sensibility of especially the posterior part of the body was diminished. Extensive disease of the spinal cord, medulla oblongata, and cerebellum was found, there being an infiltration of round lymphoid cells like leucocytes. Areas so infiltrated were abundant in both the grey and white substance of all parts of the cord, the distribution varying much. The infiltration was in the form of ramifying tracts corresponding to the course of the vessels and was probably leucocytal. Some of the nerve-cells were very granular, others surrounded by lymphoid cells. Some had a granular centre and ill-defined boundary, and in some many vacuoles encroached on the protoplasm; these vacuoles are possibly of some pathological significance. A similar infiltration of the medulla and cerebellum, but slighter, was found. In each case the effect of section of the spinal cord was tried; in the slighter case the movements continued for a few moments after pithing, in the other artificial respiration was kept up and no movements occurred in the parts below the section. This is not in accordance with the results of other similar experiments. The only morbid appearance common to the two cases was change in the nerve-cells of the cord; this is probably primary, the vascular changes and infiltration being secondary; whether the infiltration results from vascular disturbance or is due to overaction of the cells is uncertain. This detailed account of a careful examination of the central nervous organs in chorea by competent observers, and with elaborate modern appliances and methods, fills a gap in the pathology of the dog. Its result is not altogether satisfactory; it amounts to the conclusion that in chorea we find granular degeneration of the nerve-cells, atrophy of the central organs. The cessation of function in these cells may be evanescent, due to something deleterious in the blood, for Dr. Harley has produced chorea artificially in the dog by administration of the alkaloid cryptopia; the clonic spasms came on about half an hour after administration of the drug and ceased only when it was eliminated. Treatment must be essentially directed to supporting the system of the animal and determining the flow of blood to the brain and spinal cord. The latter process in acute cases may be accomplished by blisters along the course of the spine, or the insertion of a seton either in the region of the loins or in the poll. Asafœtida doses have been given with benefit in this stage. Blaine advocates the cold bath and Hill the hot; enemata are certainly useful. The iron salts are beneficial, especially in the more confirmed cases, and cod-liver oil may be given as a nutrient tonic; but nitrate of silver (half grain) and strychnia (one tenth grain), long continued and given with caution, are the only agents likely to benefit in confirmed cases. Good and carefully selected, well-prepared food must be administered throughout the attack. The prospect of recovery is best in young patients.

CRAMP is a physiological condition known as tonic spasm of a limited number of muscular fibres either of the involuntary or voluntary character. This may be a result of conditions either of the muscle, nerve, or central nervous organ. It is seen in rheumatism, in some forms of poisoning, and in dogs exposed to cold when heated by exertion or when swimming. The hind limbs are most frequently affected. It is acutely painful. The anti-spasmodic dose resorted to in such cases should consist of opium, ether, and camphor. The patient should be put in a warm bath and afterwards wrapped up in flannel. The cramp soon disappears, but is liable to recur. A timely dose of alcohol and local friction will be beneficial. Dogs liable to cramp should be kept in dry warm kennels.

TETANUS, as Blaine shows, is extremely rare in the dog, and that thoughtful comparative pathologist pertinently remarks that this is an extraordinary fact considering the liability of the dog to nervous disorders. The most familiar form is the *opisthotonos* induced by strychnia poisoning, in which the limbs are rigid and quivering, the jaws fixed, often biting the tongue, the back spasmodically curved so that the head and tail are elevated and remain so. The animal is in acute agony, and the angles of the mouth retracted, giving the expression a sardonic grin. After death the body is so stiff that it may be held out straight by the tail, and it does not decompose readily. Youatt gives an account of two cases in which the body was curled to one side (*pleurosthotonos*). Both idiopathic and traumatic cases have been recorded as affecting the dog. We know as little about the pathology of tetanus in this animal as in others. Coats finds on post-mortem examination in tetanus the central nervous organs hyperæmic. In the spinal cord, medulla oblongata, pons, corpora quadrigemina, and corpora striata, a granular material around the vessels, probably an exudation. In the medulla oblongata a longitudinal vessel at the posterior part was noted as especially affected, and here, as in other parts, there were occasional hæmorrhages. In the convolutions an exudation of a yellow fluid outside the smallest vessels, the medium ones (those most affected in the cord and medulla oblongata) having mostly escaped. And with regard to treatment it has been shown that if the animal be left in a state of perfect quietude and repose he may recover, but if subjected to officious treatment he will most certainly die.

The above-described are the principal nervous disorders of the dog; those to which the nerves and the sympathetic centres are liable have not yet been made the subject of special study. Neurotomies and nerve-graftings have been performed only by physiologists for experimental purposes; they are not yet embraced within the domain of curative surgery.

CHAPTER X.—THE ORGANS OF SPECIAL SENSE.

THE EYE of the dog differs from that of the horse in several respects interesting from an anatomical point of view. The globe of the eye is almost spherical and the pupil is circular. The retractor muscle consists of four strips and thus is much less largely developed. The cartilago nictitans is much thinner and more membranous. The upper part of the margin of the orbit is ligamentous, not bony. The iris is devoid of corpora nigra, the tapetum lucidum is whitish with a blunt edge, and the retina differs to an extent in histological detail. Undoubtedly the physiology of the organ in the two animals differs materially in special points, such as refraction, focal distances, and so on. Of diseases and accidents some special forms are seen in the dog.

A form of ULCERATION OF THE EYELIDS which accompanies mange is described by Blaine. It is denoted by obstinate swelling and loss of hair. On examination minute openings are detectable, and in a long-standing case he was compelled to inject nitrate of silver solution into these; however, generally the disease yields to an ointment of the nitrate of mercury, and prevention of rubbing and scratching the eye with the foot when the eye is "watery," profuse and persistent lachrymation being present. This sometimes depends on ENTROPION, which Braun has successfully treated by excision of an elliptical portion of skin from the lower eyelid ('Thierärzt. Mittheilungen'). Williams considers *ectropion* rare in the dog as compared with entropium and always as affecting the *lower* lid. Entropium he finds frequent in pointers and setters. He speaks of *trichiasis* as frequent in dogs. Careful examination for injury to the conjunctiva, or the presence of foreign bodies between the lids, should be made; these causes being absent, examination should next be made to determine whether OBSTRUCTION OF THE LACHRYMAL DUCT is present. It is not rare, and is considered especially frequent in spaniels. There may be a slight purulent discharge against the inner canthus. This may subside after fomentations and astringent lotions, as the obstruction is generally due to catarrhal inflammation of the lining membrane of the duct, but it may be a result of entry of foreign matter. In some dogs a watery condition of the eyes is natural, being dependent on a constant laxity of the conjunctival tissue of the eye. In such, astringent eye-salves may be tried as occasionally of some benefit. Peuch tells us that Lafosse has successfully treated lachrymal fistula by making an artificial opening into the mouth. Youatt has found LACERATION OF THE SUPRA-ORBITAL LIGAMENT present in animals destroyed on account of injury.

TUMOURS ON THE CARTILAGO NICTITANS are by no means rare; they may be conjunctival or cartilaginous, interfere with the free approximation of the eyelids, are unsightly, and may produce watery eye. They are generally congenital, but may be acquired as a result of irritation or injury. They should be removed with the scissors or knife and will seldom afterwards cause inconvenience; cautic does not, as a rule, suffice for their removal.

CONJUNCTIVITIS and SIMPLE OPHTHALMIA is denoted in the dog by the ordinary signs of this disorder and may depend on foreign bodies in the palpebral fissure, injuries, stings, poisonous herbs while the animal is in cover in the case of sporting dogs (Blaine). It has been noted after sudden changes of temperature when the animal is heated from exertion, and has also been attributed to acrid emanations in kennels, and to the acridity of soap and water left in the eyes after washing. Derangement of the digestive organs is apt to result in opacity of the cornea from malnutrition. *Granular conjunctivitis* is frequently described as affecting the dog, but must be considered a sequela of perforation of the cornea by ulceration; poppy head infusions and fomentations to the inflamed eye and exclusion of light, followed by astringent lotions and cold water applications, are required after removal of the cause in so far as is possible. When the inflammation runs very high local bleeding, preferably by leeches, may be tried. Some cases, especially those associated with skin disorder, prove very obstinate, as was noted by Blaine, who found benefit from a seton in the neck. The cornea of the dog is peculiarly liable to degenerative changes in cases of malnutrition. This is best seen in the ULCERATION which occurs in some cases of distemper. When the profuse discharge has been cleaned away it is noticeable that there is a small circular depression of the cornea; it is not yet a true ulcer, and the conjunctiva remains unbroken. Later the conjunctiva and the aqueous membrane lie together until they finally give way and the humour escapes. This is followed by a rapid profuse growth from the ulcer, which has a granulating character and gradually involves the neighbouring parts of the cornea, which become opaque and vascular. Thus, a sort of fungous growth, STAPHYLOMA, is produced which is very irritable and unsightly, and has to be removed by excision, or else, in very bad cases, the eyeball must be extirpated. Staphyloma may, however, disappear gradually either without treatment or on application of nitrate of silver and the cornea resume its original transparency; or some *opacity of the cornea* may remain. Opacity may best be dealt with by stimulation with caustic, but it often obstinately resists treatment.

DROPSY OF THE AQUEOUS CHAMBER is not rare. It is seen especially in King Charles's spaniels, and is supposed to result from an excessively saccharine diet. It is noted by undue convexity of the cornea, which also becomes clouded and gradually thinner. As the disease progresses the eye may bulge more and more until at length the cornea becomes ulcerated and the aqueous humour escapes. This result may be averted by puncture with a lancet or small trocar; there will be less chance of a mark remaining than after an ulcer. Occasionally the eye is lost after this operation from the amount of destructive inflammation set up. A seton may be inserted in the cheeks, but no cure can be effected without a radical change of diet and careful regulation of the digestive organs. The bulging of the cornea must not be mistaken for staphyloma.

TRAUMATIC DISTENSION OF THE EYEBALL results from effusion and suppuration in cases of bruise or punctured wound. Blaine obtained excellent results in such a case by evacuation with a couching needle.

The conjunctiva of the dog is occasionally the seat of DERMOID TUMOURS. The conjunctiva and skin are developed from the same source, and sometimes a circumscribed portion of the former becomes thick and bears hairs. This is generally congenital and detected soon after the young animal's eyes are opened, the attention of the owner being attracted to those organs by profuse lachrymation. The irregular part looks like a white wart, and the hairs may be seen. It varies in its degree of resemblance to true conjunctiva, and also in the amount of inconvenience it causes. It should be removed with scissors or a knife and the spot touched with caustic. Opacity may remain. Messrs. Taylor and Parker have recorded cases of this nature in the 'Veterinary Journal' for 1877; one patient was a fox terrier, the other a setter. CATARACT is frequent in the dog, especially as a result of senile changes. Thus it is almost always lenticular, and could be remedied by couching or extraction, but such an operation is manifestly open to objections in the case of dogs; the vision would not be rendered perfect by it without artificial aids, and an animal which is blind can still be petted and taken care of by a fond owner. This lesion may result from accident and then be capsular or capsulo-lenticular, but such a condition is rare. Youatt records a curious case of accidental extraction of an opaque lens by a scratch from a cat. AMAUROSIS is more often seen in the dog than the horse. It may generally be traced to blows or other injuries, such as fractures of the skull or to direct overtension on the optic nerve in cases of dislocation of the eye. It has also been seen as a senile change, but in other cases cannot be traced to any special cause. Treatment is very unlikely to be followed by benefit in confirmed cases, but nux vomica may be tried; in recent cases, especially in young animals where it may be traced to debility, or in suckling bitches, improvement may follow administration of tonics and the removal of debilitating influences. In the pregnant bitch it may disappear after her pups have been born. Amaurosis may follow an attack of epilepsy; the effect of a seton in the poll or blistering the head may then be tried.

DISLOCATION OF THE EYEBALL is seen especially in small dogs with prominent eyes and results from injuries received when fighting, more particularly scratches from a cat. The dislocation is rendered possible by the presence of a ligament instead of a bony process above the orbit; doubtless the contraction of the temporals during anger or fear facilitates the escape. The eyelids usually remain intact, and the eyeball rests on their outer surface, giving the face a most peculiar appearance. The nerve is so stretched that amaurosis is liable to follow under any circumstances, but especially when undue violence is used in the operation of returning the ball to the orbit. This may be accomplished by cleaning it, oiling it well, opening the palpebral fissure with the left hand, or elevating the upper lid by means of the blunt end of a curved needle (well oiled) and with the right hand exerting delicate pressure and slight rotatory manipulation on the ball. In some cases even a slight slit on the upper lid will be required. This accident is liable to recur, and when protrusion has taken place several times successively sutures may be inserted in the eyelids to keep them closed temporarily. Mayhew records this accident as occurring from use of the tape when medicine was being given.

EXTIRPATION OF THE EYEBALL is resorted to in cases of protrusion with thorough disorganization, also in malignant disease. It is effected by insertion of a thread through the ball from side to side and the gradual division of the structures which retain it in position, nerves, muscles, &c. Hæmorrhage may be restrained by an antiseptic astringent plug frequently replaced; granulation also is thus promoted. The use of artificial eyes in dog practice might be tried, for beauty of the patient is often an important consideration, and well-made glass eyes do not often cause irritation. Youatt relates a very interesting *case of congenital blindness from persistence of the membrana pupillaris* in a female pointer eight weeks old. The inner edge of the iris was fringed with a greyish-white fibrous matter which rendered the pupil curiously four-cornered and very small. Six months afterwards the pupil was much enlarged and of proper shape, but in the background of the eye was a faint yellow-green light. She then showed some sensibility to light and some perception of external objects. This may have been INFLAMMATION OF THE IRIS AND CHOROID, a disease resulting in lymph deposit, generally caused by injury. We have no evidence of the occurrence of specific or gouty ophthalmia in the dog.

THE EAR.—The conchial cartilage varies much in shape and length in different breeds of dogs, and we, to an extent, find that there is a difference between long-eared and short-eared dogs in their liability to certain diseases of this part and the skin which invests it. These diseases are much less severe in the present day than formerly, although we still find both external and internal canker difficult to cure. The dog suffers from *ear-ache*, sometimes without appreciable disease, but often as a result of OTITIS, inflammation of the middle and internal ear, in other cases apparently neuralgic. The general indications of disease or irritation of the ear in the dog are a tendency to carry the head to one side, to scratch the ear or rub it against the ground, to shake the head and to flap the ear violently. When such symptoms are present and the patient suffers from fever, pain, and heat round the ear, and no external indications of disease are present, otitis may be diagnosed and general and local antiphlogistic treatment resorted to. Sometimes symptoms like those of epilepsy are induced by this disorder; such violent cases were seen more frequently in days gone by, when cankers of the ear were treated with powerful irritants, than now, but I have notes on a case where post-mortem examination showed extensive suppurative disease of the bony walls of the internal ear.

Deafness is well marked in some dogs, either the result of congenital want of development of the auditory nervous apparatus or from a blocking up of the auditory canal as a result of disease. This latter condition is a not very rare sequela of internal canker, and it may also arise from the growth of tumours. Temporary inconvenience of this nature results from the turgescence of the skin caused by inflammation of the ear. A form of disorder, resulting from too low "cropping" or amputation of the conchial cartilage, consisted in retraction of the divided ring of skin into the auditory canal and union of the granulating edges, whereby the cerumen became enclosed and sometimes abscess took place. In the present day such close cropping is seldom resorted to ; it was considered useful, especially for bull-dogs, to prevent their antagonists using the ear-flaps to hold on to during fighting. The operation of cutting the external ear is resorted to still by dog fanciers, but the canine surgeon will practise it only when it is rendered necessary by disease. Peuch describes the process of amputation by the scissors or the "pince limitative."

INTERNAL CANKER is specially defined as an inflammation of the skin of the inner surface of the external ear, but it is generally associated with external canker when that disease is present. It owes its special characters to the fact that the ceruminous glands are affected in cases where the canal is invaded, and hence a red or almost black matter oozes from the external orifice; to the swollen skin blocking up that opening and rendering the escape of the discharge gradual and painful; to the fact that the parts are made much worse by the tendency of the animal to constantly shake the head and to flap the ears, causing them to ulcerate, and by the difficulty in applying agents for curative purposes to the affected skin lining the canal. This disease is first denoted by redness of the inflamed skin, this is followed by eczematous eruption and a drying of serum mixed with blood on the surface, next ulceration takes place and the formation of pus. In neglected cases fungating excrescences grow in the ear, and tend, by coalescence, to obliterate the auditory canal; the hair becomes matted by discharge, and beneath it sinuous ulcers may form and terminate in very severe ulcerative disease of the face. Occasionally there will be no eruption on the skin detectable, simply swelling around the root of the ear, and slight oozing of purulent material, and a little gurgling when the root of the ear is manipulated. The causes are accumulation of water in the ear, and (Youatt says) the determination of blood to the head from swimming in cold water; thus it is described as most frequent in water dogs; it occurs especially in long-eared animals, particularly those which are plethoric, have been confined much and highly fed. Soapsuds left in the ear after washing, accumulations of dirt, and extension of cutaneous irritation in mange also give rise to it. *Treatment* comprises keeping the patient from water, confining his ears by means of a special ear-cap such as will be described shortly, regularly cleansing the parts and dressing them thoroughly with agents adapted to allay cutaneous irritation and ulceration. Medicaments of an astringent character are preferred. Unguentum calamine is most valuable. A seton in the neck or poll, sometimes recommended, will hardly be found necessary except where the mischief is very deep seated. According to the amount of care in dressing the case will be the rapidity of cure. Coculet's treatment consists in applying a blister over the external surface of the ear by dressing every second day with tincture of cantharides $4\frac{1}{2}$ parts, tincture of galls 1 part. This allays itching and causes pain, so the animal ceases to shake his head and the disease soon heals.

EXTERNAL CANKER affects the lower margin of the earflaps; it first appears as an eruption and ulceration rapidly occurs, the skin thickens and the ulcerative change involves the cartilaginous substance. Thus the margin of the ear becomes irritable and swollen, and the disease exhibits a considerable amount of obstinacy. It is by some thought to always result from a bruise when the animal shakes his head, especially from blows of the ear-flap against the collar. It is observed most frequently in smooth-coated, long-eared dogs, and may be a concomitant of internal canker. In this disorder the collar should be left off, the ears confined with a cap, and antiseptic astringent dressings applied frequently to the diseased parts (of these a solution of corrosive sublimate has been found most effectual). In very severe cases the process of *amputation of the ears, rounding, or cropping* may be tried, the skin of the edges of the excised parts being brought together by sutures. The exposed edge may take on unhealthy action; especially does this occur when the excision has been too near the inflamed part. The *cap*

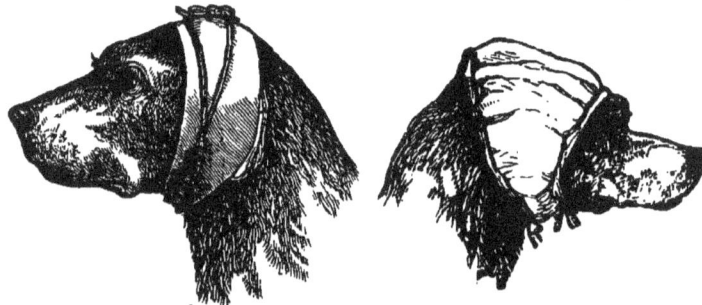

FIG. 66.—Cap for ears (PEUCH and TOUSSAINT). FIG. 67.—Cap for Ears (MAYHEW).

used to confine the ears is either the French béguin, "a kind of double pocket with four strings," or the ear bandage, consisting of two triangular pieces of cloth, united by their bases above on the nape of the neck, and each having a pocket for an ear. There are six strings, the two upper ones looped for the passage of the middle ones. All four of these pass under the jaw and are tied on the poll. The inferior pair passes crosswise over the forehead and they are tied over the nose (Peuch). Hill's ear-cap is shaped and fastened like a horse's head-piece, Mayhew's is of calico, with a tape along each margin, the tapes being

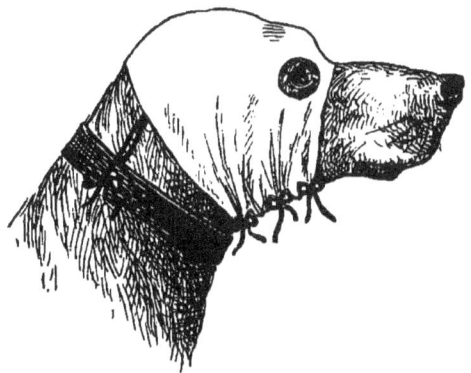

Fig. 68.—Cap for ears (Hill).

tied below the jowl. This is the simplest and best form of cap, and most easily prepared.

TICKS IN THE EAR must not be mistaken for canker; they are especially prevalent in hot countries and affect the free margin; they should be constantly and carefully removed and the parts dressed with oil of turpentine. They often cause much irritation. *Scurfiness of the flap of the ear* may arise from this or from dirt; the part should be daily washed with soft soap and warm water, then dressed with glycerine or vaseline.

SERO-SANGUINEOUS ABSCESS OF THE EAR-FLAP or *Hæmatoma* is a very painful swelling which appears suddenly, causing a tense swelling on the inner surface of the conchial flap. It results from injury and is aggravated by shaking of the head as an indication of pain. *Treatment* consists in incision along the whole length of the tumour, thus giving free evacuation to its contents, which are a blood-clot in addition to the fluid; unless this be evacuated the tumour recurs. After free incision and thorough evacuation, touch the edges of the wound with nitrate of silver (Hunting), keeping the wound open and dressing with tincture of myrrh, also protection of the ear with a cap. Mayhew takes hold of the ear and opens the part of the tumour which is then uppermost with a lancet, and then slits up the whole length by means of a probe-pointed bistoury. Trinchera after incision cuts off a piece from the edge of the wound to prevent too rapid healing, or snips out a triangular portion from near the centre with rowelling scissors ('Veterinary Journal,' vol. i, p. 63).

AURICULAR ACARIASIS has been introduced to the notice of the profession in England by an article in vol. xv, No. 86 of the 'Veterinary Journal.' It seems that Mégnin found in sporting dogs severe anæmia, epileptiform seizures (which occurred generally while at exercise), and frantic and almost continuous shaking of the ears, which caused them to die after months of suffering. He observed covering the external auditory canal a thick layer of sooty-looking cerumen, in which on microscopical examination acari, *Chorioptes ecaudatus*, were found. These parasites infest the ears of cats and other carnivora. Five per cent. solutions of sulphide of potassium frequently injected into the ear cured the patients. Nocard observed the same disease in sporting dogs which were quite deaf in many cases and were affected with epilepsy when excited in a run. The symptoms were sometimes so violent as to be mistaken for rabies and the dogs destroyed accordingly. The derangement could be conveyed from dog to dog by transfer of infested cerumen; the acari were not found in healthy dogs' ears. They are supposed to give rise to a reflex kind of epilepsy allied to the spinal epilepsy of Brown-Séquard, or to " Menier's disease " as seen in man. The following formula of an acaricide is recommended by Nocard:—Take of olive oil 100 parts, naphthol 10 parts ; sulphuric ether 30 parts. Keep in a well-stoppered bottle. Inject some of this daily into the ear and plug it with cotton wool for ten to fifteen minutes afterwards to prevent evaporation.

Under the heading *polypi of the ear* are generally described growths in the external auditory canal such as result from internal canker; these are fibro-vascular if superficially placed and cartilaginous if deep. They are probably merely the result of internal canker, not the cause of it, as was supposed by Dr. Mercer ('Veterinarian,' 1844), who in his description of them gives a good account of the ravages of the disease to which he supposed they give rise. Their surgical removal is recommended by Hill, who, like Youatt, quotes the paper from the 'Veterinarian,' *in extenso*.

THE SKIN.

The study of skin diseases in the dog has long remained empirical even to a greater degree than other branches of canine pathology. Blaine first, in this country, threw a little light on the subject in describing "Mange" as of five forms, the scabby, the red, ulceration of the sebaceous glands, surfeit, and acute erysipelatous mange. When he wrote, the influence of animal parasites in the genesis of skin diseases was just beginning to be recognised. Youatt also mentions this latter influence, but, as usual, closely follows Blaine's description of the disease, while differing from him as regards treatment. Mayhew distinguishes between parasitic mange and four other forms, of the pathology of which he was not well assured although acquainted with them practically. J. A. Nunn, in the 'Veterinary Journal,' vol. vi, published an excellent practical article on the skin diseases of the dog (which he had prepared some time before), in which scabies, follicular mange, eczema rubrum, and the diseases due to vegetable parasites, are differentially diagnosed. W. Hunting has dealt with several skin diseases of dogs in an excellent manner, his article on follicular scabies in the 'Veterinary Journal' having brought that disease prominently before the notice of the profession in England. Fleming deals with the parasitic affections of the skin in his 'Veterinary Sanitary Science and Police.' Extraordinary ideas have been held as to the anatomy of the skin of the dog; certainly this animal does not perspire so freely as most other animals, but he *does* perspire perceptibly under extreme exertion, and some of the emergencies of disease and histology has shown that sudoriparous glands exist. They open *into the hair-follicle* above the sebaceous glands, but at some distance from the epidermis. The erector pili consists of elastic fibres and white muscle-cells running from an elastic network around the hair bulb to the surface of the cutis, where they spread out and intermingle with the fibres there (Stirling). The sebaceous glands are large and well developed. The skin is specially liable to disorder in the absence of strict attention to correct hygiene; dirt, deficient exercise, too high feeding, are common sources of simple disorder, as well as predisposing influences as regards parasitic diseases. *Foulness of the skin* specially results from high feeding and want of exercise, and the animal may smell strong and look unhealthy, without any actual disorder being present. This state of affairs may be corrected by thorough cleansing, vegetable diet being gradually substituted for animal, and liberal exercise given, otherwise it soon becomes a true surfeit, or inflammatory state of the skin.

SIMPLE ERYTHEMA, or congestion of the skin, precedes actual dermatitis; it is diffused or circumscribed redness which especially affects those parts of the skin where the sebaceous glands are well developed. It occurs in association with derangement of the alimentary canal, such as may result from cutting the teeth, worms, or improper diet. It must be met with salines and cathartics, and generally proves of minor importance. A little desquamation of cuticle takes place, and the affected parts resume their normal condition. Some change should be made in the diet in cases of erythema, and if at all irritable, the affected parts may be dressed with solution of sulphate of zinc.

ECZEMA, or vesicular non-parasitic eruption on the skin, is true *dermatitis* or *surfeit*. It assumes the acute or chronic form, and is one of the most frequent diseases of the dog. It is distinguishable from the parasitic inflammations of the skin only by the use of the microscope in many cases, although a fairly accurate diagnosis may be arrived at by its macroscopic characters. Thus it is sudden in its appearance and acute, generally associated with digestive derangement or found in very young dogs after distemper, or in bitches after pupping. It especially affects sporting dogs, and follows exposure or sudden cooling of the surface of the body when heated. In the local form it generally affects the top of the head, neck, and back, but in the general form it occurs all over the body, under which circumstances the thin skin inside the thighs, on the belly, and inside the arms is found heightened in colour, and shortly the hair falls off either in moist patches or from almost the whole of the body, leaving the animal bare. The patches are dark in colour and present vesicular eruptions either spread broadcast or coalescing to form vesicles of considerable size. As the vesicles burst the watery fluid from them trickles down and dries on the surface, either forming a sort of scurf or matting the hair. This discharge is acrid, and, as Nunn points out, may putrefy in the hair, causing the extremely putrid smell of the affected animal if neglected in this stage of the disorder. During the progress of the disease the dog suffers much from irritation and causes ulcers and sores of various kinds by biting, scratching, and tearing himself in every possible way. These sores become chronic and obstinately resist cure, especially when they occur in the bends of joints. Thus in long-continued cases the lesions of the chronic disease are found; they range from a scurfy state of some part of the skin (*pityriasis*) to hypertrophy of the cutis (*psoriasis*). In this latter state the skin is thick (scurfy or with thick cuticle), devoid of hair, puckered up into abnormal folds, between which often lie sluggish ulcerated cracks. The affected parts are insensitive and very unsightly. A local psoriasis, forming elbow pads, callosities on the buttocks, and dry, thick, hairless patches on other parts specially subjected to pressure, is often seen in old watch-dogs kept constantly chained up in kennels. *Treatment.*—In acute cases the animal should receive a laxative dose followed up by salines. When he is debilitated a course of tonics may be tried, and the Liquor Arsenicalis is especially advocated. The diet must be thoroughly examined and changed when necessary, and the animal generally requires a reduction in nutritive value of the food and increased exercise. Oatmeal, meat food, and badly prepared or inferior dog biscuits are common causes of this affection which require attention. The irritation of the skin may run so high in some cases as to give rise to acute fever, which must be specially dealt with. The indications for local treatment are thorough and frequent cleansing of the body, and the control of the inflammation by astringent dressings, as the ointments of sulphate of zinc, alum, or tannic acid, according to the severity of the case. In some cases the local irritability may necessitate fomentations with opium infusions. In very young animals, cod-liver oil may be administered as a nutritive and the surface dressed with camphor ointment. In chronic cases, whether psoriasis or pityriasis be present, but little can be done likely to result in permanent benefit. Any sluggish ulcers should be dressed with nitrate of silver and calamine ointment may be applied over the affected skin. Mercurial ointment is sometimes used, but requires great caution lest it be absorbed or licked in and induce mercurialism, one of the symptoms of which, indeed, is a form of eczema occurring chiefly on the limbs and scrotum (Gamgee). At times, under climatic influences or in accordance with disorder of the digestive organs, parts of the skin chronically diseased become irritable in the extreme, and the animal can scarcely be restrained from tearing himself in his attempts to get rid of the tormenting sensation; this PRURITUS must be combated with opiate fomentations, and, if these prove unsuccessful, with the application of external stimulants, more or less powerful, according to the severity of the case. The clinical features, causes, and treatment of eczema rubrum, " red mange," or dermatitis have thus been dealt with *in extenso* because the parasitic skin disorders are actually dermatites varying in special characters, range, and extent according to their respective causes.

ALOPECIA, or baldness, is natural to some breeds of dogs, such as the polygar of Southern India. It results in all breeds from complete or partial destruction of the hair-follicles in various forms of skin disease, as ugly patches, on which the coat *may* again in time be made to grow by the frequent application of weak ointment of cantharides.

VERRUCÆ, or warts, are circumscribed hypertrophies of the papillary layer of the dermis, either congenital or the result of dirt, or growing without any distinct cause. They are often in the dog seen on the mucous membranes of the mouth and prepuce where those membranes present some of the characters of true skin. They may be found on almost any part of the true skin, but especially affect the eyelids, margins of the ears, and the lips. They can be removed by excision or the application of caustics. The warty growth which sometimes appears on the front of the eye seems to be specially frequent in the dog.

DROPSY OF THE SUBCUTANEOUS AREOLAR TISSUE, ANASARCA, is in the dog seen as a result of debilitating affections or local irritation. It is, however, rare in this animal, and principally occurs below the jaw and belly. It requires no treatment other than that for the disease on which it depends.

An acute inflammation of the skin, especially affecting the head or scrotum, has been described by some authors as *erysipelas* of the dog. Its effects extend deeper and its course is more violent than eczema; it accordingly needs more active treatment, both general and local, than that simpler form of disease. It tends to extensive sloughing of the parts or death from irritative fever, and is, fortunately, but rarely seen. It most frequently affects the scrotum (which see). Laulanié has noticed, associated with the presence of *Demodex folliculorum*, a disorder which he terms *cutaneous tuberculosis*.

PARASITIC AFFECTIONS OF THE SKIN in the dog are numerous and of much importance. Some are due to animals which permanently take up a residence at the surface of the host, others to those which are only temporary visitors. The former class of ectozoa comprise the mange dermatozoa, scarcoptes, dermatodectes, symbiotes, and acarus; the latter fleas, lice, ticks, and other insecta, such as harvest bugs. After dealing with the diseases and inconveniences resulting from these animal parasites, we shall have to note those organisms of the vegetable kingdom which have clinical importance as giving rise to ringworm and favus.

ANIMAL PARASITES OF THE SKIN (DERMATOZOA) AND THE DISORDERS TO WHICH THEY GIVE RISE.—These disorders are essentially inflammations of the skin, a fact which must be constantly kept in mind in dealing with them practically. Although they are due to the parasite, and essentially depend on its presence and activity, it cannot be doubted that certain states of the constitution and defects in hygiene predispose to the various forms of mange. So much is this the case that mange has been considered hereditary. It has been remarked that animals confined in close kennels subjected to the acrid effluvia from urine and other evacuations; those fed high and little exercised; ill cared for, starving brutes; those dogs kept on beds of barley straw, and fed with too much meat, bad flesh, or constant salt food are very liable to suffer. Contagion is, however, the active producer of the disorder; the parasites, as a fixed contagium, are transmitted by direct or indirect contact from the affected to the healthy. Some forms of animal parasitic diseases are more contagious than others owing to the habits of the organisms which give rise to them, but we have no evidence of these disorders being infectious, although the vegetable parasitic disorders are possibly so.

TRUE MANGE of the dog is technically known as SARCOPTIC SCABIES, as being similar to "itch" of man, and "scab" of sheep, and due to *Sarcoptes canis*. This parasite generally invades the skin of the back and neck, from thence gradually extending to other parts of the body, and inducing local disorders, when it invades the eyelids, ears, and feet. Fleming describes it as first affecting the face. It causes by its ravages much irritation, so that some fever is often present at first. The patient's appetite is generally good, but he becomes very thin from the amount of irritation constantly produced by the parasite. This irritation occurs especially when the skin is excited by warmth or suddenly after eating or drinking. The dog bites and scratches himself constantly and when scratched with the finger-nail evidently enjoys it. He may be covered with sores from the wounds he has inflicted on himself when attempting to remove the irritation. Examination of the skin will show red puncta or circumscribed inflammations, each of which developes into a vesicle in the majority of cases and bursts, giving exit to a sero-purulent discharge, which, mixed with epithelial scales, forms scurfs and scabs on the skin of the affected parts. The hair is soon shed, except that here and there one persists obstinately among the disease crusts. As the disease progresses more skin becomes involved, and

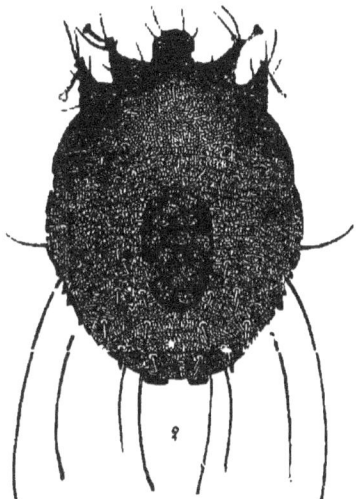

FIG. 69.—Sarcoptes canis (GERLACH).

that which was first affected becomes hypertrophied, thick, dry, scaby, and corrugated or covered with open sores from the animal biting and tearing himself. Chronic mange causes an anæmic and debilitated state of the animal, and he loses his spirits and value for sport; he is no longer keen in the field, and his powers of scent notably fail. It is observed by Nunn that the rapid spread of mange over the surface of the body is due to the fact that both bedding and claws convey the parasites. Symbiotes has been found on the dog, but sarcoptes is the general form of mange insect with which the canine surgeon has to deal. It is one of the acaridæ which burrows in the superficial layer of the dermis, and clinically may be found beneath the adherent scabs, which should be obtained quite fresh from a part which had not been washed or had dressings applied to it, preferably on a warm day or when the animal is in a warm place. The common method of obtaining the sarcoptes for examination is to place a scab under surface uppermost on the human arm; in a few hours the acarus will desert the scab and penetrate the living skin and thus give rise to a vesicle from which it may be extracted on puncture with a needle. The mange of dogs is occasionally communicated to man unintentionally and causes temporary irritation, but it is not severe and disappears spontaneously or after simple dressings, especially with Oleum Terebinthæ. Symbiotes does not apparently invade the skin of man, and therefore must be searched for by exposing the fresh crusts on black paper to the warmth of the sun's rays, when the acari leave the crusts and collect in small clusters. It must be remembered that the so-called "dry," "scabby," and "watery" manges are merely stages of the same disorder in which papules, pityriasis, or humid ezcema are present; moreover, the term "red mange" must be accepted as one applied indifferently to the sarcoptic or follicular disorder or to simple non-parasitic eczema. The latter may be present in parts of the skin of a mangy dog which have not yet been invaded by the parasites. *Treatment.*—The various methods which have been recommended by different writers on this subject, and which prove practically successful, amply prove that when treated in a proper manner and with care mange may be cured with either of a number of parasiticides. Attention must therefore be paid as to *how* medicaments are applied as well as to what special preparations are resorted to. This is a fact to be noted in dealing with all parasitic disorders of the skin where the cuticle and the scales formed on it protect the parasites from direct contact of the agent used if it be merely smeared over the surface. Therefore the animal should first be thoroughly washed with soft soap and warm water, and any hair in the immediate neighbourhood of the invaded parts cut off very close as by shaving; the scabs must be removed as carefully as possible, and the coat should not be spared if any risk of diseased parts being concealed by it be run. The smallest invaded part, if untreated, will constitute a centre for fresh spread of the disease and may cause a very considerable amount of trouble subsequently; the feet and ears should especially be examined with care lest they remain imperfectly dressed. It must be remembered in the selection of parasiticides that the dog is constantly gnawing the affected parts and also that the agents are liable to be absorbed through the sores, therefore such medicaments as tobacco and mercurial ointment, although very effectual as parasiticides, require to be used with so great caution as to be practically inadmissible, except for small patches of disease out of reach of the mouth. Whether the application resorted to be a lotion, oil, or ointment it must be applied with the greatest assiduity, well and thoroughly rubbed in, and it will require repetition at intervals not exceeding three days. Even most severe and long-standing cases will at length succumb to persistence; thus Blaine "once occasioned a very favourite setter who had had virulent mange for five years to be dressed every day, or every other day, for the extraordinary period of twelve months" before he could conquer the disease. He estimates two hours at least as the time required to dress a dog thoroughly, and when the job has been neatly managed the dog will appear nearly as clean as though nothing had been applied. He gives numerous formulæ for mange dressings, of which sulphur, turpentine, tobacco, hellebore, and tar are the active ingredients, aloes being added to prevent the dog licking them off, or the animal carefully muzzled. Mercury compounds (the nitrate, bichloride, and chlorinated salts) are advocated by him in "red mange." He gives the important practical hint that a frequent change of applications will be attended with benefit, and that the external dressings may be beneficially supplemented by a course of tonics after the bowels have been cleared out by a cathartic. The diet should be thoroughly changed, full exercise given, and the litter frequently destroyed. Hill's dressing consists of sixteen parts each of sublimed sulphur and whale oil, well blended with one part each of mercurial ointment and oil of tar. He suggests daily scalding of the kennel with boiling water, and bedding on plain straw or shavings. He uses oil of turpentine one part, whale oil six parts, ordinary sulphur ointment, and benzine or paraffin in slight cases. Mayhew applied daily, for three times, resin ointment very much thickened with sublimed sulphur and then diluted with oil of Juniper. Fleming suggests sulphuret of potassium one part, to rain water five parts, a 2 per cent. solution of corrosive sublimate in water, or carbolic acid dissolved in soapsuds (1—40), or a carefully incorporated mixture of oil of tar and sulphur, each one ounce, in a pint of common oil. His hint that "for house-dogs, and especially those with fine skins and smooth hair, a very excellent and safe remedy is the balsam of Peru, dissolved in alcohol (one of balsam to four of alcohol); this is an effective acaricide and has not an unpleasant odour," is well worth adoption. Nunn suggests for pet house-dogs stavesacre seeds digested in olive oil (1—8), and quotes Gerlach's recommendation to use creasote for short-haired dogs but decoction of tobacco for long-haired, with the comment that creasote is of objectionable odour, changes the colour of the hair, and (especially in white terriers) gives it a harsh texture. It should be diluted with 25—30 parts of oil. The decoction of tobacco should be made by pouring 25—30 parts of water on one of the dried leaves and immersing the dog for from five to ten minutes while it is still warm. Gamgee applied twice or thrice, at intervals of a day or two, the following : Creasoti 1½ parts, Sp. Vini Rect. 15 parts, Aquæ 11—14 parts. It is unnecessary here to supplement the above formulæ, which will quite meet the peculiarities of different cases and serve for periodical changes of applications as required. To summarise : change of diet, improved hygiene, thorough cleansing and disinfection of kennel, and thorough destruc-

THE ORGANS OF SPECIAL SENSE. 235

tion of litter periodically, alterative tonics after a cathartic dose, careful cleaning and thorough dressing of the skin with a suitable acaricide application, and the adoption of measures to prevent contagion are the methods to be resorted to in treatment of true mange.

FOLLICULAR MANGE is less contagious, less amenable to treatment, and less irritable than the sarcoptic form. It originates in patches especially about the head and over

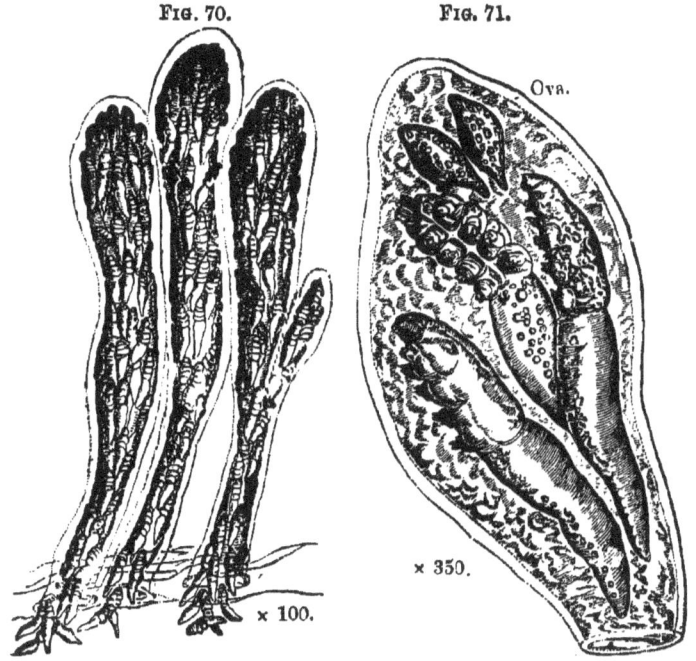

FIGS. 70, 71.—Parasites in skin follicles of dog, Follicular Scabies (WILLIAMS).
(After GRUBY.)

the cheeks and lips, but invades the whole body, especially the legs, belly, and sides, rendering the patient a loathsome object. There is more suppuration in this disorder than in true mange; the sebaceous glands and hair-follicles are the habitat of the parasite, and the latter is characterised by a large abdomen, very short legs, and great powers of proliferation. It resembles the familiar *Demodex folliculorum* of the skin of man, and possibly the two are

236   THE DISEASES OF THE DOG.

identical in species, for Gruby has transferred the disease from man to the dog and *vice versâ*. However, the specific identity has not yet been established. The obstinacy of this disease is accounted for by the remote position of the parasites and their inaccessibility, because of

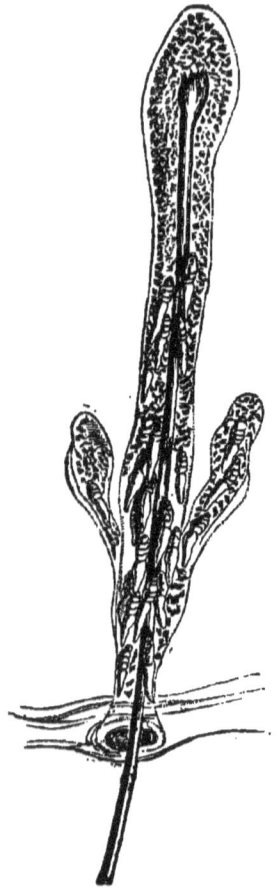

FIG. 72.—Acari folliculorum around the hair, in its follicle also in the sebaceous *culs-de-sac* (GRUBY). × 100.

the depth of the follicles and the sebaceous nature of their contents. It has been noted as of diagnostic value that in the follicular disease the body smells most offensively, and that the dog thus affected shakes rather than scratches himself, and objects to the diseased parts being handled, instead of experiencing pleasure from it, as in the true mange; in the former disease there is a burning pain of the skin, and the constitution of the patient suffers more severely. The loins, and, in the male, the genital organs, are favourite seats of the disease. Positive diagnosis depends on detection of the parasite by microscopical examination; a few strong hairs persist on the diseased parts when the rest have fallen, and often a demodex may be detected on one of these hairs as extracted by means of the forceps. Again, the mixture of pus and sebaceous matter, as expressed from an inflamed gland, may be examined under a low power, and in it will be found the acari in various stages of development and their ova; the sebaceous material may be diluted with a little oil or water to facilitate their detection. Often specimens cannot readily be obtained, then this disease must be distinguished from non-parasitic eczema by its commencing locally and its gradual extension. The hair-follicle undergoes such disorganisation that bare patches may remain after cure of a bad case; it is remarkable that the disease conveyed to man from the dog disappears after from a fortnight to a month, whereas that from man to the dog was found by Gruby to spread until the whole body surface was invaded. The earliest indication of this disorder consists in circumscribed loss of hair and the occurrence of red spots, of each of which the opening of a sebaceous gland is the centre, serum forms, and subsequently rather large pustules, which burst, and their contents form scabs. The pustules are often confluent, and the skin of the affected parts is much inflamed throughout. The patient suffers much, and the loss of hair may be so extensive as to render careful clothing of the animal necessary in cold weather. Cracks and other sores form on the surface, and sometimes blood from them mingles with the purulent discharge. *Treatment.*—The general rules which we have propounded for the treatment of parasitic mange must be remembered and applied here as in "true mange." The local treatment needs to be specially active, because the parasites occupy a position which prevents the immediate access to them of the dressings which are resorted to. Therefore the latter should contain some alkaline substance, especially potash, as has been pointed out by Hunting and Duguid, which acts on the epithelial tissue of the skin and probably saponifies the fatty matter of the sebaceous and hair-follicles. Hunting's dressing is olive oil, fourteen parts, shaken up well, with one part of creasote and then two parts of strong Liquor Potassæ added, to be applied every third or fourth day to all diseased parts with a piece of rag, the dog having been washed a few hours before each dressing. Zurn uses ointment of benzine (1—4); Weiss inunction with essence of juniper; Zundel Ung. Argent. Nit., or Ung. Hydrarg. Verd.; or Balsam of Peru, one part dissolved in alcohol, thirty parts (Fleming). Mayhew recommends a mixture of equal parts of nut oil, spirits of turpentine, and oil of tar, which may be applied after washing the body carefully with a strong solution of carbonate of potash. Hill prefers mercurial dressings. Remove all hair of affected parts by clipping or shaving; Hunting insists on this on the grounds that the presence of hair encourages the growth of the parasites. Thus the treatment of follicular mange exactly resembles that for true mange, but some dressings are found most valuable for the former and others for the latter. Constitutional treatment and disinfection must not be forgotten. Sometimes several months' active treatment is required for this disease, for agents which destroy the acari may yet not suffice to render their ova incapable of being hatched in due course and causing the disease to break out again on parts where it has apparently been cured. A bedding of red pine shavings is specially recommended by Nunn in cases of mange; it is preferable to pine sawdust, is cheap, easily procurable, does not get into sores or the coat, and it does not cake into a hard mass. Care should be taken to change it twice weekly, and to burn the old bed.

SKIN DISEASE DUE TO LEPTUS AUTUMNALIS, THE HARVEST BUG, has been described and figured by Friedberger

('Archiv f. Wissensch. u. pract. Thierh.,' 1875), also by Defranc, Mégnin, and Fleming. Kuchenmeister described the harvest bug as a human parasite causing boils, obtained in the autumn from grass and stubble. It affects animals in July and August; at other time it is supposed to undergo developmental changes in mossy places. It is frequent in countries with chalky soil, and burrows in the skin. It

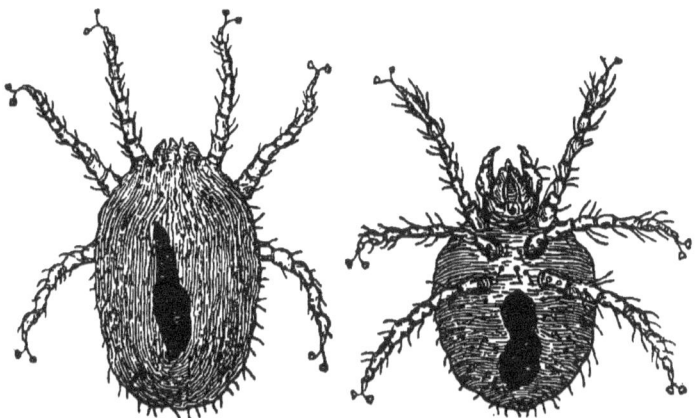

FIG. 73.—*Leptus autumnalis.* (After FRIEDBERGER.)

produces irritation, especially when the part is rubbed, which causes it to expel acrid ejecta. Before it has burrowed it may be detected with the naked eye, as its bright red colour renders it conspicuous. It most frequently attaches itself to the head or upper part of the neck or back of the dog. It causes at first a great deal of irritation of the skin and eczematous changes, indicated by the usual symptoms. In some cases there is little actual irritation but bare spots of irregularly circular form are found scattered over the head or upper part of the body. On the more recent spots the bright red parasite may be detected by means of a small hand lens. Fleming found that paraffin dressing answered in a few days, but the skin looked unhealthy for some weeks. Friedberger found that energetic washing only seemed to extend the disease; he tried the effect of 4 per cent. solution of carbolic acid in glycerine. His case had already been going on for about six weeks.

TICKS are frequent on dogs, especially in summer and in tropical countries. They debilitate the patient by suction of his blood and are most loathsome to the owner. They sometimes bring on paralysis, either directly by the weakness they cause or by reflex influences. They especially collect iu the ears. Andersen, in his 'Lake Ngami,' mentions that the bush tick found in South Africa kills dogs and even oxen. The species usually found on the dog is *Ixodes ricinus*; it should be removed with forceps, or each individual cut in two and the skin dressed with a little turpentine. In other cases mercurial dressings may need to be resorted to with the usual precautions.

FLEAS, *Pulex irritans*, collect on the dog in large numbers and cause very severe irritation; it is not uncommon in India to see dogs in an advanced state of debility, apparently the result solely of the number of partial parasitic pests (fleas, ticks, and lice) roaming about in the coats. As, also, fleas prevent pet dogs being nursed, a satisfactory method of extirpating them is a desideratum. Washing the animal with soft soap and water, or with carbolic soap, should be carefully performed, and then while the animal is yet wet, his coat should be thoroughly cleaned with a small-toothed comb. As Blaine points out, the preliminary washing is necessary to enable the comb to overtake the parasites. The dog should be allowed to sleep on yellow deal or red pine shavings, and the skin periodically dredged carefully once or twice a week with either powdered sweet flag (Acorus Calamus or Bussumboo), powdered camphor, or finely powdered resin mixed with bran. Gamgee recommends a dressing of oil of anise seed with common oil; Hill a mixture of Spts. Camphoræ with half its bulk of oil of turpentine and one sixth its bulk of carbolic acid mixed with chilled water. Various insect powders and dog soaps are advertised for the removal of fleas; some of these require to be used with the greatest caution, as also tobacco water and mercurial preparations, such as are sometimes recommended. Cleanliness of the dog and his kennel, washing the latter out with hot water and turpentine, and pine-dust bedding, frequently changed, are necessary.

LICE, *pediculi*, cause less irritation than fleas, but look much more objectionable. They affect especially certain parts of the body, such as around the anus, at the junction of the thighs, on the back, and inside the ears. They are the concomitant of dirt and can be got rid of by cleanliness strictly enforced. Mayhew suggests a dressing of the whole body surface with castor-oil. Hill prefers the ammonio-chloride of mercury, either as a powder brushed into the coat, or as an ointment applied thoroughly and left on for five or six hours, the animal being muzzled during that time.

THE DERMATOPHYTIC DISEASES OF THE DOG, or those due to vegetable parasites, are two in number of importance from a clinical point of view. The general principles which guide us in the treatment and prevention of animal parasitic diseases of the skin apply also with regard to these disorders, but it is found that some agents are specially well suited to destroy vegetable parasites, and that the latter spread much less rapidly than animal parasites and cause much less irritation and constitutional disturbance. The vegetable parasites are fungi, and, as such, are mainly made up of spores and hyphal elements; they invade the epithelial constituents of the skin, and consequently we find that in the vegetable parasitic diseases fungal elements may be detected in hairs examined under the microscope. These diseased hairs often are obstinately retained in position while all around are shed and they are enlarged and friable, breaking off irregularly. The dermatophyta especially prevail in damp weather, ill-drained kennels, and among young animals, also the absence of cleanliness and want of sufficient food predispose, but contagion is essential to communication of the disease. The parasite may be obtained from other species than the dog, and may also be transmitted to other animals, such as mankind. The communication may be mediate or immediate, and evidence tends to support the belief that the spores of pathogenic fungi may be transported through the air. The nidus of growth somewhat affects the characters and habits of the fungus, especially as regards luxuriance; thus St. Cyr has shown that the dog is particularly liable to favus. It has been stated that the ringworm fungus of the dog has larger spores than that of the horse, does not disappear from the skin spontaneously, and will not develope on the ox, although that of the ox readily developes on the dog. The incubation of these vegetable parasites varies from eight days to a fortnight; they belong to the genus Achorion *v.* Trichophyton, and the disorders to which they give rise are termed Tineæ. They are not frequent in the dog nor severe, and readily yield to treatment. Fleming relates a case ('Veterinary Journal,' vol. i, p. 207) in which it was obtained from a horse.

TINEA TONSURANS *v.* RINGWORM is not common in the dog; it was first noticed as affecting that animal by Gerlach. It is denoted by circular patches, devoid of

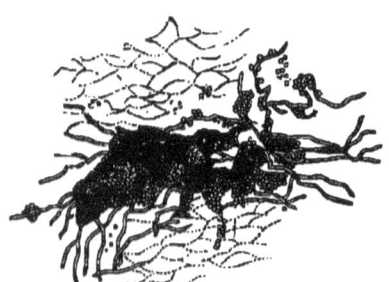

FIG. 74.—*Achorion Lebertii* (FLEMING).

hairs, except a few enlarged broken ones which persist. These patches grow at their margins and so may become confluent; they are shiny in appearance and covered with glistening scales of epithelium or with a greyish crust. The hairs and epithelial scales of the affected parts contain *Achorion Lebertii v.* Trichophyton tonsurans. The disease readily yields to improved hygiene, constant cleansing with soap and water, and dressing with tincture of iodine, mercurial ointment, acetic acid (glacial), tincture of cantharides, Unguentum Argenti Nitratis, sulphurous acid lotions, and many other substances, either of which will prove successful in removal of the parasitic disorder if carefully applied. This disease must not be confounded with herpes circinatus, a non-parasitic disease in which vesicles form over small circular patches, especially in young dogs. As a result of teething or indigestion herpes is rare and soon disappears spontaneously.

TINEA FAVOSA *v.* FAVUS *v.* HONEYCOMB RINGWORM differs from the above in the habit of growth of the fungus, *Achorion Schönleinii v.* Tricho. favosa, which gives rise to it. This parasite, when it has gained contact with the surface of the body, enters the hair-follicle and developes in and about the hair. At first it causes a slight epithelial proliferation around its base, then the hair (itself diseased) becomes the centre of a cup-shaped crust of a sulphur yellow colour. In advanced cases these crusts become confluent and form an ugly shapeless tumour, sometimes of enormous size, consisting of fungal elements and causing absorption of the tissues against it by pressure. The mass smells like cat's urine, and usually grows on the head of the dog, such being probably the result of the dog catching the disease from affected mice. In treatment all affected hairs and favus crusts should be carefully removed, *not* with the finger-nail, and destroyed by fire; the exposed

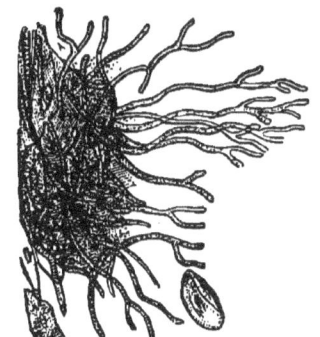

FIG. 75.—Achorion Schönleinii in early stage of development, mixed with epithelial scales (BENNETT).

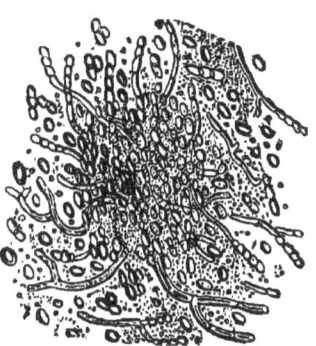

FIG. 76.—Achorion in more advanced stage from centre of a favus crust (× 300). (BENNETT.)

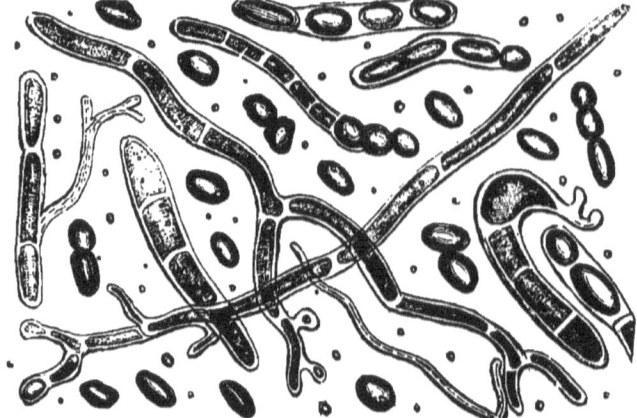

Fig. 77.—Thalli, mycelia, and sporidia of Achorion (BENNETT). × 800.

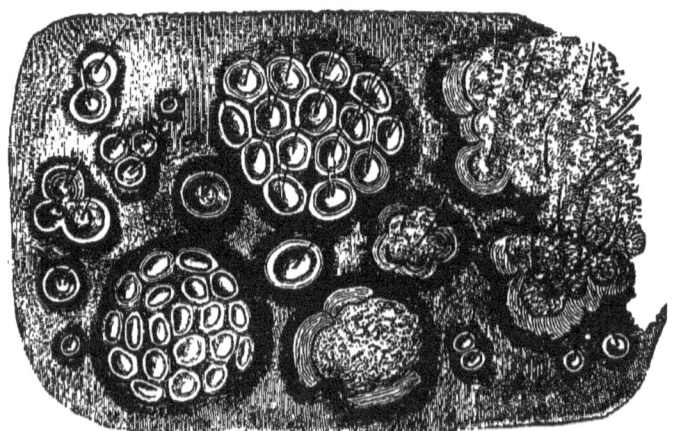

Fig. 78.—Tinea favosa crusts in various stages (BENNETT). Natural size.

parts should be thoroughly washed and the diseased surface thoroughly dressed with one of the applications suggested for ringworm, preferably corrosive sublimate solution or the ointment of nitrate of silver.

CHAPTER XI.—THE LOCOMOTOR SYSTEM.

THE bones of the dog are light in build, but strong and with well-defined processes. As the union of epiphyses with the shaft occurs some considerable time after birth it is not rare to find apparent fracture from a breaking through their cartilaginous bond of union. This must be always remembered in dealing with very young animals, in which especially fracture is liable to occur. Repair under these circumstances is effected with remarkable rapidity, indeed by the simple process of normal bone formation; care is, however, required to ensure proper direction of the limb during union of the parts.

TRUE FRACTURE is very common in dogs, as they are very liable to blows and to injuries of various sorts, as when they are run over by a carriage or fall from a considerable height. The small size of dogs enables us to manipulate their limbs when injured freely and to reduce fractures and dislocations such as in the horse, for instance, would be quite incurable. The fact that dogs are very clever and careful in saving injured limbs is also in favour of securing repair. Diagnosis is generally very simple from the abnormal mobility of the injured part, and from the clear and well-defined arrangement of the limb muscles and bones. Crepitus, deformity, and, later, inflammation, are detectable. The causes of fractures in dogs are direct violence, as blows, kicks, falls from a moving carriage or from the high window of a room in which they have been shut, and so on. The bones of the limbs are the most frequent seat of injury, but cases are on record of fracture for almost every bone of the body. In variety, treatment, and processes of repair these injuries to the skeleton of the dog differ in no respect from those of other animals.

However, we may advantageously note *seriatim* some of the principal fractures of the dog and examine their special features.

The *skull* is small, rather deficient in processes, and the two halves of the lower jaw are movable on one another. These facts render fractures of it infrequent. When the *walls of the cranium* give way after falls or blows, compression and concussion of the brain have to be considered and dealt with, and depressed portions of bone removed by trephining and elevation, and the further progress of the case is apt to be complicated by meningitis. There are two points strongly in our favour in treatment of dog fractures, that there is seldom much constitutional irritation and the reparative powers are very rapid. These must be considered in prognosis. The *lower jaw* may be fractured by blows, as a kick from a horse, or may simply be dislocated at the symphysis. Such cases generally recover spontaneously, although loose teeth or fragments of bone may need removal by operation. The *vertebræ* may be fractured when an animal is crushed by a door slamming to or by a carriage wheel passing over him; dislocations and incurable paralysis is liable to result. *Fractured ribs* may be associated with fatal pleurisy or lung perforation; generally these bones act mutually as splints; they are very elastic in the dog on account of the length of their cartilages, an anatomical peculiarity which protects them to an extent from being broken. When that accident occurs a bandage may be put tightly round the chest to limit the respiratory movement of the ribs and the animal kept quiet. *Fractured pelvis* acquires special importance as liable to cause impediment to parturition when it occurs in bitches. It may prove so much so as to necessitate delivery by Cæsarean section. The *scapula* generally gives way in the region of its neck, although fracture of its blade is not infrequent from kicks and blows. The mobility of the part is limited by a pitch plaster, perhaps strengthened with splints of pasteboard or wood, and the shoulder retained against the side by some such device as a starch bandage embracing the neck and forearm like a figure-of-

THE LOCOMOTOR SYSTEM. 247

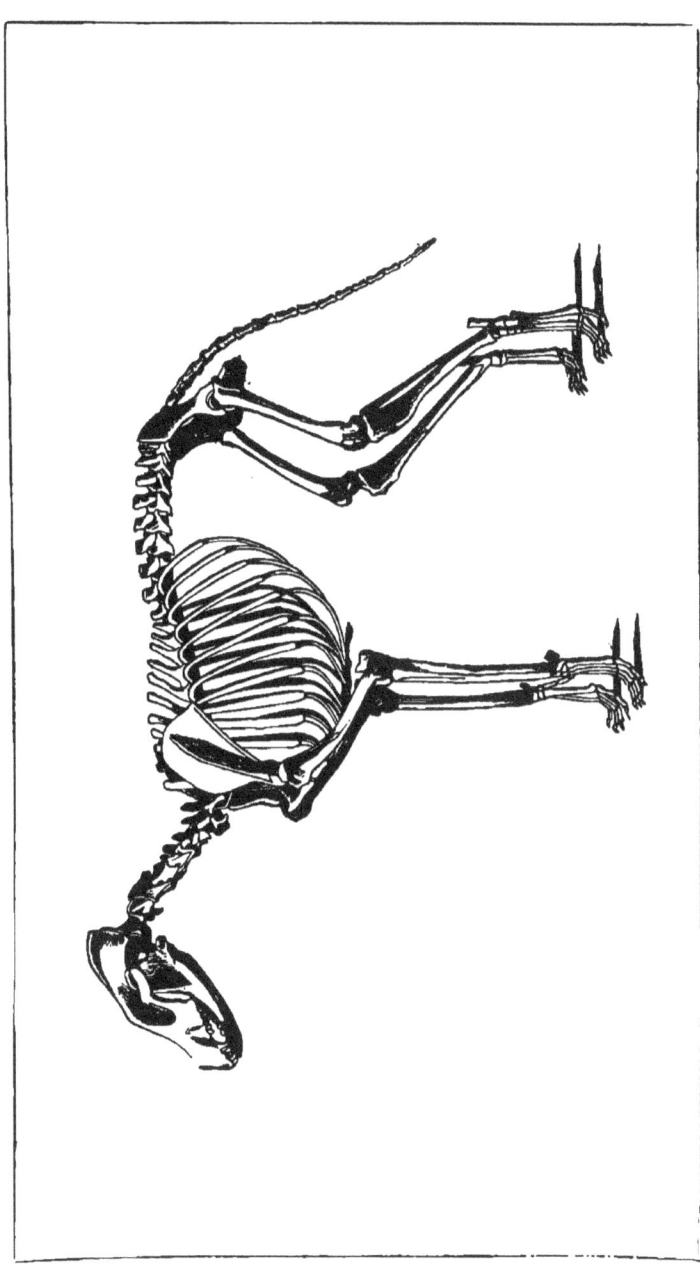

FIG. 79.—Skeleton of dog (CHAUVEAU).

eight, and then brought several times round the girth and back. The *femur and humerus* are among the bones most frequently fractured, but the *radius and ulna* or *tibia and fibula* give way still more often. In the case of either of these bones the limb should at once be tied up firmly with a handkerchief, whereby displacement may be prevented or lessened, and as soon as the necessary appliances can be procured the parts snould be " set," and retained by means of splints and bandages. The " setting " must be effected by extension and counter-extension, the splints may be of gutta percha, pasteboard, pliable wood, leather of moderate thickness, or sheepskin. These must be retained by bandages arranged in special adaptation to the requirements of the case, which generally necessitates considerable ingenuity in order to allow for the necessary amount of swelling and to prevent displacement such as is very liable to result from the movements of the patient, especially when the injured bone is painful from the reparative changes going on in it. Pitch, starch, gum solution, or plaster of Paris are used to render the bandages and splints firm, and enable them to give the necessary support to the limb without shifting. They are smeared over the injured part or bandage, or the latter is steeped in them just before application. The splints may be rendered more pliable in adaptation to the form of the limb by soaking in warm water, but, especially at their ends, they should not exert undue pressure on the skin so as to cause ulceration. The bandages, too, must be put on with judgment, allowance being made for the subsequent swelling of the injured parts. Blaine's means of treatment of fracture of the thigh consists in the application of a pitch plaster spread on moderately firm leather to the outer side of the thigh, and extending a little over the inner side also. Attaching to this a long splint such as will extend from the toes to an inch or two over the back, to be retained by a long bandage carefully put round the limb from the toes upwards, and continued up the thigh, it must then be crossed over the back, continued round the other thigh, and fastened. It must be kept from slipping over the tail by means of another slip passed round the neck and along the back. ('Canine Pathology.') The same method is applicable in fractures of the shoulder. In fracture of the femur, Peuch straps the thigh up against the belly, and keeps the rest of the limb stiff with a bandage; he also insists on the necessity of bringing all splints to the end of the limb to prevent gangrene. Mayhew describes and illustrates his method of setting and retaining fractured legs. He brings the divided ends of the bones together and retains them as follows. Three broad straight ribbons are cut from a stout sheet of gutta percha and are soaked in warm water

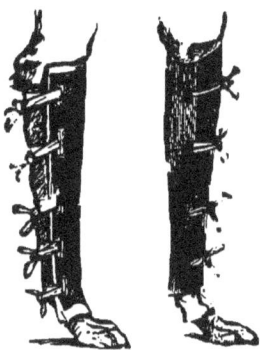

FIG. 80.—Method of setting fractured legs (MAYHEW).

until they are pliable, several holes, resembling button-holes, having been cut in them first by the aid of a punch and a narrow chisel. "When they have lain in water a sufficient time to soften, and no more, for the water of too great a heat shrivels up as well as softens the gutta percha, he draws forth one ribbon, and this he moulds to the front of the sound leg. That done, he takes another piece of the putta percha, and this he models to the hind part of the sound leg. The remaining slip is fixed to the side of the limb. After the pliable gutta percha has been forced to assume the shape desired, it is covered with a cloth saturated in cold spring water which hastens the setting of the material, and thus shortens a process which renders the dog somewhat uneasy. The splints are then braced together and fixed on the limb by means of a long piece of tape, a quantity of lint, to protect the soft tissues, being put under them. The tapes are run through the holes previously made and wound round the limb over the splints not too tightly at first." *Fracture of the metatarsals or metacarpals* may be complete, when the foot is crushed and all four bones have given away, or incomplete, when the uninjured bones will act as splints and materially hasten the healing process. The crushed foot will require to be supported by splints. When a toe is crushed it is generally best to amputate it. Splints should be kept on for at least four weeks in order that the callus may become sufficiently consolidated to support weight, otherwise a FALSE JOINT may form, the fragments being united by fibrous or cartilaginoid material instead of true bone. This unsatisfactory result is most frequently seen in ill-nourished animals, especially those of rachitic tendency. A seton may be passed through the imperfect union, or the repair may be begun over again by its surgical division; the patient should receive good nutrient food and lime-water doses. It is sometimes necessary to break through the callus recently formed, when the union is such as to render the limb permanently bent; the bone must then be reset, and the case treated as a recent fracture. The refracture, as being very painful, should be performed under chloroform. A muzzle should be put on after the setting of a limb, and the animal kept as quiet as possible. A cathartic dose is useful to prevent excessive inflammation.

DISLOCATIONS assume a more important place in the history of the dog than in that of the horse or ox. Their treatment is very similar to that of fracture, with which they are not infrequently complicated. This is seen especially in the *elbow-joint*, where the inner condyle of the humerus becomes separated, and the limb is found flexed inwards. Occasionally outward dislocation occurs at the elbow. When, as is generally the case, this lesion occurs in a young animal, it is difficult to detect crepita-

THE LOCOMOTOR SYSTEM. 251

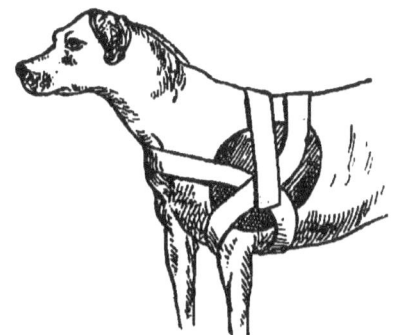

Fig. 81.—Bandage for fractured scapula (Hill).

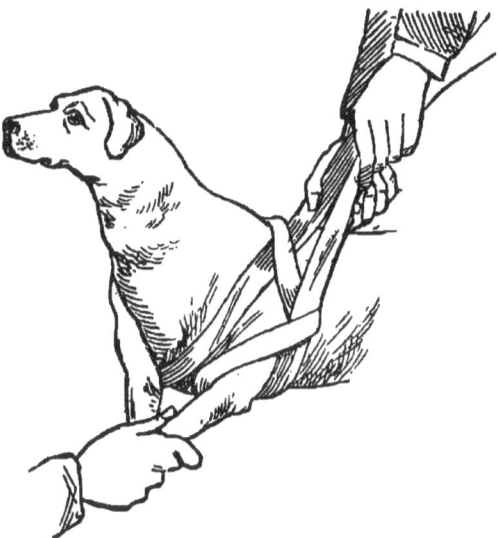

Fig. 82.—Dislocation of shoulder-joint (Hill).

tion, but fracture may usually be correctly diagnosed. Peuch and Toussaint remark that the "horse and dog are the only animals in which humero-radial luxation is observed." *Dislocation of the shoulder* sometimes occurs, and may be reduced by extension and counter-extension. Hill accomplishes this easily by passing a strong towel or surcingle underneath the brisket, between the forelegs, over the withers, round the girth, and across the front of the breast. This is held firmly, while an assistant steadily draws the limb in the direction required. The *knee* and *hock* also, are liable to dislocation. The *patella* is not infrequently "put out;" it may be restored by pressure while the foot is held forward, and retained by a bandage. The *coxo-femoral joint* is liable to dislocation in the dog, in which animal it is rendered possible by the absence of a pubic-femoral ligament and by the length of ligamentum teres. In its reduction, in addition to extension and counter-extension, a certain amount of rotation will be found necessary. The *small joints of the foot* are sometimes "put out" by injuries. Lafosse has recorded three cases of *luxation of the lower jaw* of the dog, a very remarkable lesion and scarcely possible without fracture, considering the firm hinge-like union between the bones and the smallness of the interarticular cartilages. Bandages, splints, and adhesives may be applied for dislocations as for fractures, and care must be taken lest the injured joint be used too early, before thorough repair has occurred. Blistering or application of the hot iron may be needed to complete the cure.

ANCHYLOSIS AND EXOSTOSIS is referred to by Blaine as follows: "*Stiff joints, splints*, and *spavins* occasionally enter the kennel as well as the stable, and when not too far advanced in the ossifying process may sometimes be checked by a blister repeatedly applied." Peuch and Toussaint recommend firing superficially in these cases, and allude specially to exostoses of the elbow, stifle, and hip. These diseases are most frequent in sporting dogs, as also are SPRAINS, ranging from extensive subcutaneous rents in muscle, or the "breaking down" of sinews (espe-

THE LOCOMOTOR SYSTEM. 253

cially in greyhounds), to slight wrenches of joints such as disappear on application of cold water combined with rest for a couple of days. These injuries must be treated on exactly the same lines as those of the same nature affecting the horse. A remarkable form of *laceration of the trapezius muscle* occurs in carnivora, especially in cats. It is denoted by the upper part of the scapula ascending considerably above the withers when the weight is thrown on the limb.

The Foot of the dog, although not nearly so often the

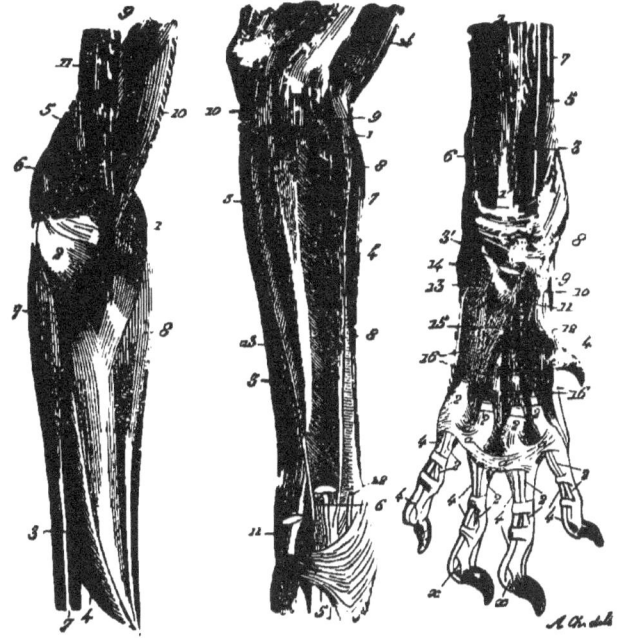

Inner face of forearm.   Outer face of forearm.   Posterior surface of foot.

FIG. 83.—Muscles of forearm and foot of dog (CHAUVEAU).
(For names of different structures indicated by letters and small numbers
'Chauveau's Anatomy' must be referred to.)

seat of lameness as that of the horse, yet suffers from some disorders of importance. In cases of lameness traceable to the foot the animal generally carries the diseased part in the air, and when at rest licks it frequently. When such signs are present it is necessary to make a thorough *examination of the foot.* The cutaneous balls or "pads" should be examined for suppuration, especially apt to be due to thorns and injuries. Also they are liable to be too much worn by a long day's march or hunting over hard rocky ground. The possibility of the foot having been crushed or contused must not be forgotten. The claws should be carefully looked to for overgrowth or sinuous ulcer, and between the toes we may seek for parasites or injury; sprain, dislocation, and fracture may occur in the foot. SORE FEET may be *overworn*, when they are tender but recover in a day or two after bathing with sulphate of zinc lotion, or, as a domestic remedy, milk. They should be wrapped up carefully in poultice cloths or protected by a leather boot. *Foundered* feet are those in which inflammation of the true skin has occurred. It is generally the result of too long journeys, and indicated by high fever, inflammation of the balls of the feet with suppuration, and even exposure of the sensitive layer so that the animal cannot stand, suffers acute pain, and constantly licks the part. This disease is especially seen in sporting dogs which have had too little exercise out of the season and are suddenly brought into work; it also results from contusions on rough ground and from exposure to cold, as "frost-bite." The changes induced may produce permanent soreness of the feet and so render the animal quite unfit for future work. Such cases may best be dealt with by fomentations and poultices if the animal will allow them to remain on. The foot should be protected with a boot, and febrifuge medicines and a laxative dose will tend to promote a cure. This disease is very liable to recur, a fact which should be carefully remembered. In some cases of *mange* the root of the claw is affected by the ravages of the parasites, ulceration takes place, and the horny appendage becomes quite loose. The disease is obstinate and resists ordinary remedies, and does not seem to be improved by the animal almost constantly licking it. The claw may in this case be removed, after which the remedial agents will act directly on the diseased parts, and cure will rapidly be effected;

while this is taking place the foot should be protected by a boot. *Sinuous ulcer underneath the claw* is generally denoted by an oozing, sometimes so slight as to be only with difficulty detectable, from between hair and claw, generally through a small orifice against the lower part of the claw. This has been found in some instances to result

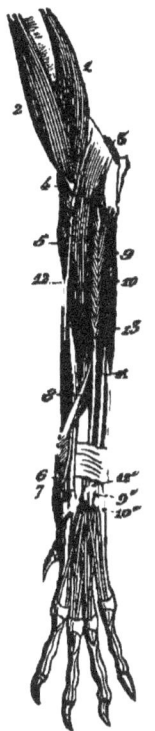
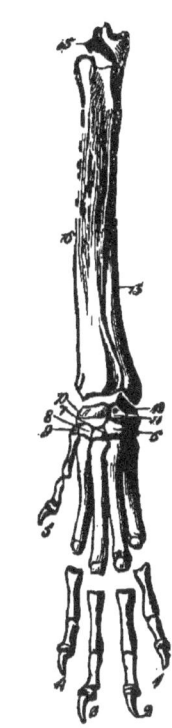

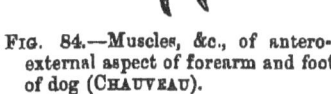

Fig. 84.—Muscles, &c., of antero-external aspect of forearm and foot of dog (CHAUVEAU).

Fig. 85.—Bones of forearm and foot of dog (CHAUVEAU).

from the use of sand on the floors of kennels. In such a case the horn must be removed so as to open out the ulcer; the foot should then be poulticed, and after it assumes healthy action be dressed as a common wound. In bad cases the claw must be completely drawn, which will not be difficult as it is already much undermined by pus accumulation; it will be reproduced but imperfectly. *Thorn wounds of various kinds*, and other such lesions require no special notice here. *Overgrown claws* are directly associated by Mayhew with a life on Turkey carpets and silk dresses. Hence they are generally seen in small animals which seldom have to run any distance. The unworn toenail curls in the direction of a ram's horn, and it may penetrate the balls of the foot and cause extreme pain and suppuration. It must be removed by means of a small triangular saw, or the rowelling scissors used for the horse, or else a stout pair of wire nippers. The two latter instruments are preferable to plain scissors, for the latter is liable to split the horn, and to the saw because its operation is long and sometimes painful.

AMPUTATION OF THE TOE* is performed by the flap method, as described in detail by Mayhew. The one most frequently removed is the inner of the hind foot, which is quite rudimentary, its metatarsal having degenerated into two diminutive articular extremities and a central fibrous shaft. These "*dew-claws*" are sometimes simply clipped off with scissors, in other cases they require more systematic amputation. The reasons for their removal are three : the liability of their claws to overgrow and do mischief, their sometimes injuring the opposite leg when the animal is running fast, and their being apt to catch in tangled bushes and so on, in cover. Thus their removal is useful and justifiable, in fact an absolute necessity in the case of sporting dogs.

PARASITES BETWEEN THE TOES worry the animal extremely by giving rise to constant irritation which sometimes causes him to tear the skin of his feet savagely.

CONGENITAL DEFORMITIES of the limbs are not infrequent in puppies. Perhaps that most often seen is due to malformation of the lower end of the humerus which presents two rounded condyles; of these one rests on the radius as usual, the other on the ulna. The effect of this

---

* For an intetesting case of amputation of the toe for encephaloid of the second and third phalanges of the forefoot of a retriever see 'Veterinary Journal,' Oct., 1885.

is that the elbow-joint, partially or entirely, loses its ginglymoid character, and cannot support the weight of the body, so it yields under the animal. An interesting case is recorded by Wolstenholme ('Veterinary Journal,' xi, p. 342). The patient was a five weeks' old, silver-haired, terrier, dog puppy. Each forearm was twisted from the elbow, so that the radius along its entire length was on the ground. The anterior surfaces of the carpi met and touched, from which point the fore paws were sharply turned outwards, with their plantar surfaces at right angles to the ground. The outer surface of each humerus was concave to admit the displaced elbow; progression was difficult. The patient was healthy, but, of course, the deformity did not admit of cure. In cases of congenital malformation or acquired contraction of tendons, *tenotomy* has been successfully performed on the dog. The flexors of the foot are not infrequently thus divided; and Peuch mentions successful section of the external and oblique flexors of the metacarpus some distance above their insertion into the subcarpal bone.

CANCEROUS DISEASES OF BONES, as also OSTITIS, PERIOS-TITIS, and other simple diseases present no special features in the dog; Bouley and Faugré have amputated at the shoulder-joint in incurable lesion of the limb; the patient remained useful as a watch-dog.

CHAPTER XII.—POISONING.

ALTHOUGH this subject constitutes a special branch of science known as toxicology, to works on which the canine pathologist must refer for information as to the effects of excessive doses of medicinal agents and for the phenomena associated with the ingestion of poisons as detectable ante- and post-mortem, there are several practical aspects of poisoning which must be noted here. It must also be remarked that as dogs have been the animals most readily available for experiments of a physiological, therapeutic, and toxicological nature, so there remains scattered through the works of Christison, Orfila, Majendie, and many more recent scientists, an enormous amount of information which, when carefully digested, will be of great value to the canine pathologist, but which, it must be confessed, would have been even more valuable if the experimentalists had obtained a sounder acquaintance with the phenomena of natural disease in the dog. Some very remarkable facts have been ascertained about the action of remedial agents on dogs. Thus Orfila has remarked that whereas opium injected as enema or intravenously is narcotic, it is not so on gastric ingestion. Henbane has been noticed as specially powerful in its action on dogs. CARBOLIC ACID is of especial importance in its toxic action on carnivora, which renders it a dangerous application in canine practice. When used extensively over the skin, or to wounds, or when taken internally, either by licking or as administered medicinally, it produces immediate depression, weakening of the heart, convulsions, and speedy death, the blood being found tarry in consistency and colour; the carcase has a tendency to mummify rather than decompose. Carbolic acid may be safely resorted to as an external application for dogs in the form of ordinary carbolic soap, or the following preparation, suggested by Broad of Bath, may be used. Take of No. 5 carbolic acid and of soft soap equal parts, and of water one pint to the ounce of both of the ingredients. Boil the pint of water until the ounce of soap dissolves, and then add the ounce of acid, and, as soon as the boiling point is again reached, set aside; dilute to 1—40 for local application, to 1—50 for general application, for dogs. The same writer recommends in cases of carbolic poisoning continuous application of cold water by means of a watering pot with the rose on, until the convulsions cease ('Veterinary Journal,' vol. iv, p. 261). The skin should be thoroughly cleansed with cold water and hard soap, or oil well rubbed over the surface; stimulants should be given internally.*

Tobacco Water and Hellebore solutions used externally in skin diseases may be similarly absorbed or ingested, and cause serious depression or even death. Such agents should be used only when the animal can be kept under close supervision, where the skin is not much abraded, and when a leather or perforated tin muzzle can be applied. If the animal seems depressed or vomits, he should be at once thoroughly washed in a cold bath, which will prevent absorption and thoroughly dilute the poison. MERCURY COMPOUNDS, such as the Unguentum Hydrargyri, when licked in, may give rise to acute ulceration of the bowels, with profuse diarrhœa and bloody evacuations, prostration, and death. *Eczema mercuriale* is an effect of ingestion of mercury, or its incautious use externally, which has been especially noticed by Gamgee. The animal is dull, off feed, breath and skin secretions offensive, and profuse salivation is also present. The hair falls off in herpetic patches, found especially inside

* Kunde in carbolic poisoning gives castor-oil with some aromatic stimulant and saccharate of calcium. His formula is—water, 50 parts; sugar, 15 parts; slaked lime, 5 parts. Mix, and shake every half hour for some time ('Gaz. Méd. Vét.,' 1874).

the legs and on the scrotum. Professor Bennett, in his 'Principles and Practice of Medicine,' gives some interesting figures of the bones of a dog which introduced much mercury into his system by licking vermilion paint. Numerous cancerous-like masses were found in the lungs and internal viscera, and the skeleton had undergone most remarkable changes in the long bones, mainly of the shafts, *not of their extremities*. "The disease closely resembles what may be observed in many other specimens of so-called syphilitic disease, yet in this dog we have the

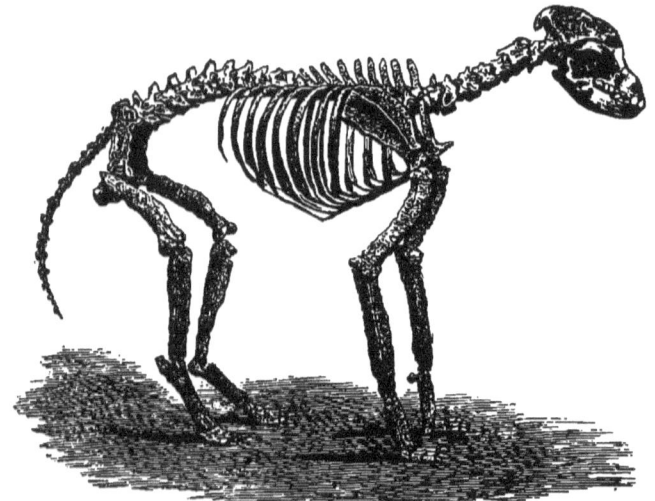

Fig. 86.—Skeleton of dog. Effects of mercury (WILLIAMS). (After Professor BENNETT.)

positive proof that it was caused by mercury, as all attempts to communicate syphilis to dogs have failed."

Vegetable poisoning is not common in the dog; the toxic agents from which he suffers are generally mineral, and picked up accidentally or intentionally with meat or other animal substance. Hounds are liable to suffer from poison, either as intended for destruction of foxes or actually designed to destroy the pack with a view to "boycotting" hunting. Poison intended for cats or for various kinds of vermin may be eaten by dogs;

verdigris may be taken in deleterious doses by consumption of stale food out of brass vessels. Corrosive sublimate, arsenic, or verdigris thus ingested produces very violent vomiting, diarrhœa, and acute inflammation throughout the alimentary canal. The vomits and alvine evacuations are laden with blood. Blaine considers ulceration of the mouth with extremely offensive breath, when found with the above symptoms, conclusive evidence that corrosive

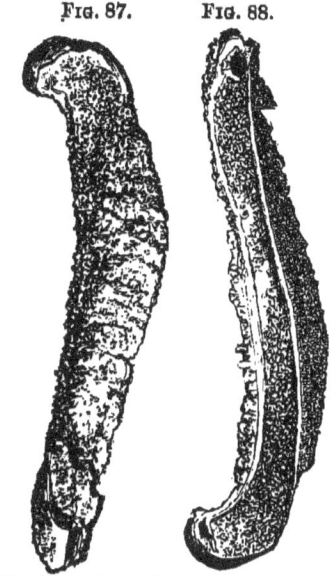

FIG. 87.   FIG. 88.

FIGS. 87, 88.—Two views of the femur. Effects of mercury (WILLIAMS). (After Professor BENNETT.)

sublimate has been used. In all such cases the nature of the vomits should be carefully examined, and they should be, if necessary, analysed. They may contain portions of the skin of the animal used as bait. The first vomit needs special attention. Early detection of the true nature of the poison may enable us to give an antidote in time, but in all such cases liberal doses of milk, white of egg,* or

* The white of one egg is required for every 4 grs. of the poison (Peschier). Iodine and acetate of lead are considered the best counter-agents for mercurialism.

blood serum should be given. Cases of convulsions from ordinary pathological conditions and various other diseases are liable to be confused with irritant poisoning in hasty diagnosis.

Strychnia when used as a poison may be determined by the tetanic convulsions to which it gives rise, the straightness of the back, elevation of the tail, rigidity of the limbs, and sardonic grin on the countenance, the symptoms appearing suddenly. Valenti, of Kino, saved twelve dogs after overdose of strychnia by means of monobromide of camphor in small doses (4—6 grammes) given by the stomach. The action of the antidote is sure and rapid in reducing the force and frequency of the spasms, which become clonic instead of tonic, the hyposthenic action of the bromide mitigating the reflex activity of the strychnia. The bromide acts on the sympathetic nerve inducing myosis and cardiac paralysis, and, if an overdose be given, it and the strychnia together produce death by syncope. If the latter only causes death the cardiac impulses continue post mortem ; this is not so when the bromide is the cause of fatality ('Veterinary Journal,' iii, p. 51). Young animals are less susceptible to the action of strychnine than adults, herbivora than carnivora. Feser, of Munich, finds that of the 1 per cent. solution of nitrate of strychnia one milligramme subcutaneously, and five to six times that amount by the mouth per kilogramme of the weight of the animal may be given as a medicinal dose. In the 'Veterinary Journal,' vol. xi,* Butters, of Norwich, relates a case of successful treatment of strychnia poisoning in a retriever bitch. She was kept under the influence of chloroform for one hour, then given extract of belladonna gr. xij in solution, Tinct. Opii ʒj, and received chloroform, with occasional intervals and doses of ten minims of hydrocyanic acid occasionally, for two hours, when the belladonna and opium was re-

* In a case of strychnia poisoning recorded in vol. vi of the 'Veterinary Journal,' chloroform relieved the tetanic convulsions, being given five or six times in three hours. No spasms occurred after this, and the next day the dog seemed quite well though dull and stupid.

peated. The spasms at last ceased, leaving her weak and prostate, but she was all right again the next morning. Post mortem in these cases the body is found very stiff, remains so for some time, decomposes slowly, and there is a diffused yellowness of the tissues; the muscles are of a specially bright colour.

Lead-poisoning is mentioned by Blaine as resulting from the animal lapping water from the leads of buildings, or eating paint. It is denoted by vomition, colic, and vertigo, followed by paralysis, and must be treated by administration of sulphate.

EUTHANASIA, or a speedy, sure, and painless death, one not likely to hurt the feelings or brutalise the thoughts of the operator and lookers-on, is a great desideratum as regards dogs, because it is necessary as a measure of sanitary police to limit the number of stray and useless dogs, dangerous to the public as liable to convey rabies, and prevented by the excellent sanitary conditions of modern West of Europe towns from obtaining a well-earned living by scavengering, as do the dogs of Constantinople and most Oriental cities. Dr. Richardson has especially studied the best method of slaughter, and considers that *carbonic acid poisoning* is to be preferred to all others, the gas being liberated by chemical means in a chamber in which the dogs are confined. *A powerful electric shock* is equally effectual, but requires more elaborate appliances. *Drowning* is a speedy death, and not painful, but it is offensive to the feelings, and the same may be said of pithing, destruction by a blow on the head, and hydrocyanic poisoning. A dose of *prussic acid* causes death in a couple of minutes, but the fatal result is preceded by struggling and convulsions, which, however, are not indicative of pain. Of ordinary prussic acid from a freshly opened bottle half an ounce to an ounce should be given to prevent accidents, although much smaller doses would prove lethal; it is as well to leave a margin for individual peculiarity of constitution and for accident, also care should be taken to ensure that the victim is thoroughly dead, for cases have been known in which an animal, supposed to have been killed, has subsequently been found running about the room, having expelled the poison by vomition, or outlived its sedative action. It is wonderful how long an animal may have been apparently dead from prussic acid poisoning, and yet be revived under the influence of ammonia.

SNAKE-BITE is a form of poisoning sometimes seen in England from the viper and adder, but it is very common abroad, and proves rapidly fatal. The dog suffers great distress and rapid decomposition of the blood; the injured parts swell, and all control over them is lost; convulsions early set in. The best treatment is ligature by tourniquet above the punctures if a limb is injured, prompt cauterisation if possible, or local and general administration of Liquor Ammoniæ, full doses of the agent being given half-hourly. Cold affusions and artificial respiration may prove of benefit. It has been proved that if artificial respiration be kept up long enough, the action of *curara, wourali, or the Indian arrow-head poison*, whereby it paralyses the respiratory centre, will pass off, and the animal's life be preserved. This poison has the remarkable power of paralysing the motorial apparatus in such a way that the animal suffering from it, if operated on, has no power of showing its agony by movement. It is expressly forbidden to be considered an anæsthetic under the Act for the regulation of vivisection.

The stings of wasps, bees, hornets, and other insects may even prove fatal to dogs, aud hunting dogs are especially liable to suffer from accidentally disturbing nests of these creatures. Water affords the best means of escape, dense smoke also keeps off the irritated insects, a thick bush may afford some defence. Indigo in the form of vegetable blue-ball (as used for domestic purposes) is considered an excellent application for wasp and bee bites; ammonia locally and generally is required in some cases, carron oil will be found useful in others, but often, especially when a hornet's nest has been disturbed, the dog will die before assistance can be rendered.

CHAPTER XIII.—MINOR SURGERY.

TUMOURS.—In treating of the diseases of various organs we have noted the occurrence of different sorts of tumours in or on them. The system of the dog seems especially liable to morbid growths, which not rarely assume the MALIGNANT FORM. Cancers seem to specially affect the genitals and the mammary gland, and are most frequently scirrhous in character, although epithelial cancer and encephaloid are, perhaps, most frequent in the dog of all our domesticated animals. It is found that over-fed, under-exercised, and old dogs suffer most from cancers, and hence, in their removal, when chloroform has to be resorted to, the greatest care has to be exercised lest the heart be fatty; probably the effects of local anæsthesia might be more frequently relied on than they usually are in canine surgery. There is an increasing belief that many tumours of the genitals and elsewhere in the dog are less frequently malignant than is generally supposed, but as the use of the microscope has extended among veterinary surgeons the frequency of morbid growths in carnivora has been thoroughly established. *Melanosis* is very rare, but Fleming has placed on record an instance of disease of the skin of the leg which proved to be " Black Cancer," and on post-mortem examination the liver and heart were found the seat of black deposits. *Sarcomatous growths* of the limb bones are sometimes seen in the dog ; in the ' Veterinary Journal,' vol. viii, is recorded a case of osteosarcoma of the femur of a cat.*

* Quite recently Rivolta, the illustrious Pisa professor, has detected in the masses of diffused sarcoma of a dog, a form of mucedo, which fungus he terms *Micorimyces canis familiaris.*

Of NON-MALIGNANT GROWTHS, *fibrous or fibro-vascular polypi* are very common, and occur in the nasal chambers, rectum, vagina, and even on the sheath. *Simple fibroma* follows injuries, and is most frequently found on the limbs. *Fibro-cystic tumours* occur on various parts of the limbs, especially on the toes, and in the form of " capped hock " and " capped elbow," which are common in dogs kept in small kennels without sufficient exercise. They result from bruises, and abscesses may form, but generally they are a kind of spurious bursa, and covered by skin much hypertrophied, and with thick horny cuticle.* Similar spurious bursæ form in certain breeds of dogs opposite the tubera ischii from the animals constantly sitting on hard ground. They resemble the " natal callosities " found in monkeys.

Warty growths, simple epithelial hypertrophies, are common on the skin and mucous membranes, as of the sheath and mouth. Acetic acid is a good caustic for them, and Blaine recommends that they be dressed with a powder consisting of equal parts of savin and sal ammoniac powdered.

Fatty tumours occur in and on the skin or in the subcutaneous tissue in certain breeds of dogs, such as spaniels, very frequently. They especially affect old animals, and may be freely removed with the knife, being generally well defined and lobulated, also loosely connected with the subjacent parts. Blaine speaks of the frequency of formation of fatty tumours in the region of the loins of spayed bitches. It appears as a swelling on each side of the loins, and is simply fat accumulation at the seat of the ovaria. *Osseous growths* occur usually as exostoses, which have been elsewhere mentioned, but osteoids have been described as lying independently in the soft tissues, and occasionally tumours in the mammary gland undergo calcareous or osseous change.

* Lowe reports an interesting case of cystic growth at the lower part of the cervical region. It recurred three times after operation, and finally disappeared on removal of much of the investing integument ('Journ. Comp. Med. and Surgery,' iv, p. 317).

The various tumours, malignant and non-malignant, found in the dog, must be treated on ordinary surgical principles.

WOUNDS, too, will present no special difficulties to the surgeon. In most dogs they result from bites, and special care must be taken lest they be poisoned with rabid saliva. In the absence of this complication they may be poisoned by foulness of the mouth of the animal which inflicted the bite, or of the patient himself, which latter affects the wound if he be allowed to lick it. Dogs recover in a most marvellous manner from injuries of extraordinary severity, often without any treatment, but in neglected cases maggots may form and the wounds become most offensive, as, especially, in the neglected stump of an amputated tail. As regards treatment it has been found that stitches are especially liable to ulcerate out rapidly in the dog, and it must be remembered that carbolic dressings must not be applied to his wounds so freely as to those of most other animals. Also he should generally be kept closely muzzled, lest, when an irritable condition of the wounds comes on at a certain stage of healing, he produce serious complication by lacerating the edges of the wounds with his teeth. In sporting dogs *gunshot wounds* are not unfrequent.* Jewsijensko has studied injuries of this nature in the dog by cruel experimentation, and his results are hardly of sufficient importance to justify his proceedings. The same cannot be said in detraction of the experiments of Professor Parkes, the results of which may be read in the 'Quarterly Journal of Veterinary Science in India,' vol. iv, No. 13, p. 97, and which throw much light on an obscure point in human surgery. The most severe wounds inflicted on dogs are generally the result of fighting, for which purpose several of the breeds are specially trained. It is a matter of no slight importance to be acquainted with the best and *safest method of separating and securing fighting dogs*. We may adopt the suggestions contained in Fleming's work on ' Rabies and

* Broad has recorded an interesting case of encysted bullet in a dog's foot in vol. iv of the 'Veterinary Journal,' p. 93.

Hydrophobia.' "The only safe place to grip a dog is at the back of the neck, behind the head; there the skin is sufficiently loose to afford a good hold, while the hands cannot be touched by the animal's teeth so long as the grasp is maintained. . . . Blows will not prevent their biting and holding on. . . The simplest, safest, and by far the most effective plan of rescuing one's self, or defending other persons or dogs from some infuriated or mad animal's fangs, is *choking*. If the animal wears a collar this is easily done, as one has only to seize it firmly at the back, and pull it tightly against the throat in front; the foot or other hand may usefully aid in the operation by pressing strongly against the back of the neck. It should by no means be released immediately it lets go its hold, but ought to be still further choked until it is harmless for the time, when means may be had recourse to for securing it properly. When there is no collar on the neck a strong handkerchief or piece of rope tied round and pulled in the same manner, or twisted with a stick, is a ready appliance. . . It only requires strong arms and a little coolness and tact."

Tabular Statement of Doses, and Special Actions and Uses of Medicines in Canine Practice.
(Mainly after Finlay Dunn.)

Name of agent.	Medicinal dose.	Special actions and uses internally.	Special actions and uses externally.
Acetic Acid	♏︎iij; vinegar ♏︎xv	To be freely diluted	—
Aconite	B.P. Tinct. ♏︎v; Fleming's ♏︎j; ext. gr. ss	¼ gr. Aconitine fatal to a 30-lb. dog in 65 minutes	—
Rectified Spirit	fl℈ss	—	—
Aloes	℈j	—	—
Alum	gr. xv	—	—
Chloralum	gr. viij	—	A dilute solution useful for mange, fleas, and ticks.
Ammonia solution	Fort. ♏︎viij; medicinal solution ♏︎xvj	—	—
Ammoniacum	gr. xv	—	—
Ammoniæ Carb.	gr. v	—	—
,, Chlor.	gr. xij	—	Used, finely powdered and mixed with an equal quantity of savin leaves powdered, for removal of warts, particularly when their situation and character are such as not to permit of their eradication by other means (Morton).
Liq. Amm. Acet.	ℨj	Well diluted (5 to 6 times its bulk of water) Specially useful in epilepsy and asthma	—
Amyl Nitrite	♏︎j	—	As an anæsthetic in vapour ♏︎j to xx (Tuson).
Anisi fruct.	gr. xl	—	—
Antimonialis pulv.	gr. viij	True James' powder a good febrifuge and diaphoretic for the dog (Simonds)	—

DISEASES OF THE DOG.

Name of agent.	Medicinal dose.	Special actions and uses internally.	Special actions and uses externally.
Tartar Emetic	Emetic, gr. ij; sedative, gr. j	—	—
Areca Nut	About ½ nut, i.e. gr. lx; i.e. gr. ij per pound weight of the dog	—	—
Arnica	♏vj	Useful in kennel lameness and stiffness from over-exertion, both internally and externally.	
Arsenious Anhydride	gr. 1/15; liquor ♏x	More active in carnivora than in herbivora	
Santonin	gr. iij	—	—
Asafœtida	gr. xv	—	—
Belladonna	Leaves gr. vj; extract gr. iij	Useful in chorea	—
Atropine	Per orem gr. 1/60; subcnt. gr. 1/120	Antidote to Morphine (Binz)	—
Buckthorn Syrup	ʒiss	Given combined with Confect. Senna ʒj–ʒij, Jalap gr. x–xv, or Castor Oil fl ʒj	—
Calabar Bean	gr. iss	—	—
Physostigmine	gr. 1/12	—	—
Quicklime	gr. xv	—	—
Lime Water	ʒv	—	—
Calcium Carbonate	gr. x	—	—
,, Phosphate	gr. viij	—	—
Calumba Root	gr. xv.	—	—
Chlorinated Lime	gr. iv	—	—
Camphor	gr. viij	Given in emulsion with eggs, or dissolved in milk or oil	The vapour of Camphor destroys fleas.
Cantharides	gr. j	—	Vesicant action weaker in dogs than in horses; stronger than in cattle.	Blistering ointment. ℞ Pulv. Canth. ʒj, Ol. Tereb. ʒj, Adipis ʒxij. Misce.
Capsicum; Carbolic Acid	gr. ij Crystals miss; Sodium salt gr. x	—	—

Cascarilla Bark	gr. xxv	—	—
Castor Beans	6 beans; oil ℥ijss	—	—
Catechu	gr. viij—xvj	—	—
Chamomile Flowers	gr. xxx	—	—
Charcoal	gr. xl	—	—
Chloral Hydrate	Per orem gr. xv; Hypod. gr. vij	Full doses produce emesis	—
Chloroform	♏viij, as antispasmodic	Repeat every 2 hours, or even oftener	—
		In weak spirit, repeated after 1 or 2 hours. "To prevent vomiting the previous meal, given 3 or 4 hours before, should be light and easy of digestion" (Dunn)	—
Chloric Ether	♏ʒj	"No tonics are better adapted for badly nourished dogs, especially when suffering from distemper; they allay irritation, counteract perverted and inordinate nervous action; given along with port wine or ether they prevent untoward complications and expedite recovery" (Dunn)	—
Cinchona Bark	gr. xxx		—
Quiniæ Sulph.	gr. iij; Cinchonine gr. vj		—
Cod-liver Oil	ʒij twice a day for weeks	"For dogs and cats it is particularly useful in protracted cases of distemper, rickets, inveterate skin disease, epilepsy, chorea, and chronic rheumatism, especially that variety known as kennel lameness, and depending upon damp, bad feeding, and faulty nutrition." (Dunn)	—
Colchicum	gr. v	Dogs are readily brought under both its irritant and sedative effects	—
Copper Sulphate	Emetic gr. viij; tonic and antispasmodic gr. j	Persisted in until it interferes with the appetite in chorea and epilepsy. Useful as a prompt emetic in narcotic poisoning	—
Cupri Amm. Sulph.	gr. iss	Useful in mange and follicular mange	Spirituous solution (1—8), useful in canker of the ear of dogs; 5—10 drops introduced daily (Simonds). Too irritant an external application for dogs.
Creasote	♏j	—	
Croton	Seeds 1 or 2; oil ♏j	—	

272 DISEASES OF THE DOG.

Name of agent.	Medicinal dose.	Special actions and uses internally.	Special actions and uses externally.
Digitalis	gr. ij twice a day; Digitaline gr. 1/16	"Valuable in dogs debilitated by distemper or overwork, as giving greater coordination and expulsive power to the ventricles, and greater tone to the relaxed capillaries, and thus renders the weakened and irregular circulation steadier, slower, and stronger. Further, it usually relieves difficulty of breathing or dropsical effusion which has resulted from imperfect action of the heart." (Dunn)	—
Dover's Powder			
Ergot	gr. x		
	ʒj; gr. ii—x (Tuson); Liquid ext. ♏vj	Carnivora more susceptible to its action than herbivora	—
Ether	♏ xl	Etherization has been maintained for upwards of an hour in dogs	—
Euphorbium			
Fern Root	ʒij; fluid ext. ♏ x; repeat in three days if necessary	A dose given fasting sometimes dislodges tænia in three hours	—
Galls	gr. viij		
Gallic or Tannic Acid	gr. iij	Useful in prolapsus ani and piles	—
Gamboge		Too drastic for dogs	Apt to cause sloughing and blemishing when applied to the skin of dogs.
Gentian	gr. x twice a day		
Ginger	gr. xx		
Glycerine	ʒiij twice or thrice daily to delicate dogs	"In dogs troubled with flatulence and acidity, glycerine given before eating is useful." (Dunn)	—
Gregory's Powder	gr. xv		
Gums	gr. xxx		
Black Hellebore			
Conium	Succus flʒj; tinct. flʒj; ext. gr. ij	"Repeated twice daily, and persisted with in quantity sufficient to paralyse voluntary motor power." (Dunn)	—

Hyoscyamus	Succus ♏xxx; tinct. ʒij; ext. gr. ij; Hyoscyamine gr. 1/16 ♏viij (dilute)	
Hydrochloric Acid		Chemical effects on the blood less marked in carnivora than herbivora
Indian Hemp	—	Effects most marked on carnivora and omnivora
Iodine	gr. iv twice a day a couple of hours before eating	Dogs are more susceptible to its action than horses or cattle
Ipecacuanha	gr. xx; Dover's powder gr. xij	"Drop doses of ipecac. wine, given at half hourly intervals to arrest vomition in weakly dogs, and for this purpose it is advantageously combined with nux vomica and morphine, while the spray is occasionally used to diminish expectoration and irritation of winter cough, and allay some forms of asthmatic dyspnœa." (Dunn)
Citrate of Iron and Quinine	gr. vj	
Ferri Carb. Sacch.	—	A specially convenient agent in canine practice
Iron Sulphate	gr. viij	Iron continuously administered contracts and condenses the spleen (Weinhold)
" Iodide	gr. iv	
" Perchloride	Of weaker solutions, ♏vj his v. t er in die	
Jaborandi	gr. xx; Pilocarpine gr. ⅓ hypod.	Causes perspiration, less in horses and dogs than in men
Jalap	ʒss	Is a good cathartic, specially effectual if combined with 1—2 grains of Calomel. A good cathartic (Dunn): ℞ Jalap ʒss—j Calomel gr. ij—iij { in holus; acts in 2 or 3 hrs. if given to a dog fasted for 6 hrs.
Juniper	Berries gr. xxx; oil ♏vj	
Kamala	ʒij	—

Name of agent.	Medicinal dose.	Special actions and uses internally.	Special actions and uses externally.
Kusso	ʒiv	—	—
Sugar of Lead	gr. iv	—	—
Linseed Oil	fʒj—ij	"For dogs, especially when young, when the digestive organs are in an irritable state, and when exhausting disease has reduced the strength, linseed oil is a very suitable laxative, and is more effectual when given with an equal amount of castor oil" (Dunn)	—
Magnesium Oxide	ʒj	—	—
,, Sulphate	—	Has no stimulant action on the liver (Rutherford)	—
Mercury with Chalk	gr. ij, 3 or 4 times a day	Used to allay gastric irritability and as an alterative	—
Blue Pill	gr. v	Mayhew's Purgative Dose: Blue pill . . . 5 grains, Powdered Colchicum . 6 grains, Extract Colocynth . 10 grains. Dunn's Purgative Dose: Blue pill . . . 5 grains, Comp. Ext. Coloc. . 10 grains, Ol. Piment. v. Ol. Caryoph., a few drops to flavour.	—
Mercury Red Oxide	—	Even a few grains produced fatal gastro-enteritis	—
Calomel	gr. ij	Three or four times a day with an equal amount of Opium. Emetic combined with an equal amount of Ant. Pot. Tart. in tepid water	—

TABULAR STATEMENT OF DOSES, ETC.

Corrosive Sublimate	gr. 1/12	—	To allay irritation of the skin apply 2 grs. Corrosive Sublimate added to 2 min. Prussic Acid, and water 1 oz. (Dunn). Corrosive Sublimate 5—10 grs. in water 4 oz., effectual in mange and for destruction of lice. Care must be taken to prevent the animal licking himself (Morton).
Methylic Alcohol	♏viij	Allays gastric irritability and persistent vomition	
Mustard	gr. xv; stomachic	A dessert-spoonful in several ounces of water a handy emetic. Oil of mustard is powerfully vesicant	
Myrrh	gr. xv		
Nitric Acid	♏viij; dilute medicinal acid	Dissolved in 80—100 parts of water greatly relieves tenderness and tension in piles	
Acid, Nitro-hydrochloric	♏iv; dilute medicinal acid		
Nux Vomica	gr. j twice daily; tincture ♏xx (B.P.)	Should be given combined with a laxative	
Strychnia	gr. 1/16	A smaller dose in proportion than that of herbivora	
Oak Bark	ʒj	Useful for piles in decoction	
Olive Oil	fʒij		
Opium	Gum gr. iij; tincture ♏xxiv	Useful in obstinate vomition, dysentery, and in strychnia poisoning. Best administered to the dog in the form of syrup of white poppies (Youatt)	
Acetate of Morphia	gr. 1/4 per stomach; gr. 1/16 hypodermically	Doses insufficient to kill excite rather than produce soporific effects	A hypodermic injection of Atropine with Morphia is useful in asthma.
Peppermint, Oil of	♏iv	Peppermint water given in ounce doses	
Peppers	gr. vj	Act violently on omnivora and carnivora	
Petroleum	—		
Podophyllin	gr. iss—v	United with diuretics given in dropsical affections	
Potassæ Tartras Acida	gr. viij	Useful for snakebite (Shortt)	
Caustic Potash	—		
Carbonate of Potash	ʒss		
Sulphuretted Potash	gr. vj	Useful in chronic cough, rheumatism, and skin diseases	

Name of agent.	Medicinal dose.	Special actions and uses internally.	Special actions and uses externally.
Potassium Sulphate	—	—	—
Iodide of Potassium	gr. x (bis in die); gr. j—v (Tuson)	—	—
Bromide of Potassium	gr. xij	Useful in epilepsy and convulsions	—
Nitrate of Potash	gr. xx	"A good febrifuge" (Dunn): Nitre . . . 5 grains, Dover's powder . . 5 grains, Calomel . . . 1 grain.	ʒj—ij added to water, one pint, effectually allays itching (Ainslie).
Chlorate of Potash (dilute) Prussic Acid	gr. x (Phar.) mIij	Valuable in gastrodynia and obstinate vomition	—
Quassia Infusion	fʒj	—	—
Resin	ʒj	—	—
Rhubarb Root	Stomachic gr. xj; laxative gr. xx; [ʒij—iij, Tuson]	—	—
Salicylic Acid	gr. x every 1 or 2 hrs.	Useful in chorea, epilepsy, and chronic gastric irritation; also in diarrhœa and dysentery (5 to 10 gr. in 1 oz. starch solution) (Dunn)	10 to 20 gr. to 1 oz. of distilled water forms a solution which destroys the parasites of mange and ringworm, and weaker solutions are sometimes used as clysters to bring away ascarides (?) from the rectum of horses and dogs (Dunn).
Savin	gr. iv		
Nitrate of Silver	gr. ¼ (chorea) gr. ss (diarrhœa)		
Soaps.	—	With water cause emesis	—
Sodium Carbonate	gr. xv		
„ Biborate	—		
„ Sulphite	gr. xx	—	In ointment useful in eczema, alternated with that of Zinc Oxide.
„ Chloride	Emetic ʒj; tonic gr. xv		
Chlorinated Soda	gr. xx	—	—

TABULAR STATEMENT OF DOSES, ETC. 277

Stavesacre	.	Infusion ℥j—Oij of water	—	Seeds boiled in vinegar yield a solution which not only kills pediculi, but also, when rubbed into the skin, destroys their eggs. A strong solution, too freely applied sometimes nauseates and prostrates delicate subjects.
Sugar	.	℥j	—	—
Sulphur	.	Laxative ℥j; alterative ℨj	—	—
„ Iodide	.	gr. viij	—	Applied externally in skin affections (Prof. Brown).
Sulphuric Acid	.	♏iv several times a day	—	—
Sulphurous Acid	.	♏xxx	—	—
Sweet Spirits of Nitre	.	fʒss	—	—
Tobacco	.	gr. vj; decoct. fʒiij	A single drop of nicotine destroys small dogs in 5 minutes	—
Turpentine	.	gr. xl; oil of, ♏xl	Oil is an antidote to phosphorus poisoning, and is "an effectual but not always safe vermifuge and purgative, being given in combination with olive oil, and in doses varying from ʒj—ʒiv." (Morton)	An occasional sprinkling over dogs' beds keeps them free from fleas. ℨj, A prompt blister:—Ol. Tereb. . ℨj, Medicinal Amm. ℨiij. Bland Oil .
Valerian	.	ʒj; Sodium, Zinc, and Iron Salts gr. iv	The iron compound most certain. Useful in chorea, epilepsy, hysteria, and nervousness	—
Valerianate of Quinine	.	gr. iij	—	—
Veratrum	.	gr. iv	Useful for the nervous sequels of distemper	—
Vaseline	.	—	—	—
Wax	.	—	—	Dogs are liable to suffer from absorption of strong dressings.
Zinc Oxide	.	gr. vj	—	—
„ Sulphate	.	Astrin. tonic gr. iij; emetic gr. x in 2 or 3 oz. of water	—	—
„ Chloride	.	—	—	—
„ Acetate	.	—	—	—

INDEX.

	PAGE
Aberrations of intellect	200
Abnormal urination	159
Abortion	186
Abscess, ear-flap	223
— jaw	103
— liver	143
Absence of œstrum	183
Acariasis, auricular	224
Acaricide	224
Accumulation of tartar	100
Achorion Lebertii	242
— Schönleinii	243
Acid, carbolic	258
— carbonic	263
— prussic	263
Acupuncturation	209
Administration of pills	14
After-treatment of parturition	195
Air passages	86
Albumen in urine	153
Albuminous nephritis	153
Alopecia	228
Amaurosis	217
Amputation, external ear	220, 222
— penis	168
— toe	256
— uterus	177
— vagina	180
Anæmia	71
Anasarca	229
Anæsthetics	20
Aneurism	81
Anidian monsters	193
Animal parasites, skin	230
Anthrax	58
Antiseptic surgery	25
Aphrodisia	184
Apoplexy	204
— parturient	205
— pulmonary	97
— splenic	151
Apparatus, generative	165, 170
— urinary	153
Appendages, fœtal	193
Applications, external	21

	PAGE
Aqueous chamber, dropsy of	216
Arctic dog disease	40
Arrow poison	264
Artificial cystic calculus	157
Ascarides	122, 132
Ascites	138
Asthma	95
Atony of rectum	129
Atrophy, kidney	155
— ovaries	171
Auricular acariasis	224
Auscultation	89
Balanitis	163
Baldness	228
Bandaging	23, 24
Barking, excessive	87
Baths	22
Bees' stings	264
Behaviour, general	10
Belly, tapping the	139
Benign variola	60
Biliary calculi	147
— fistula	147
Bilious infarction of bowels	142
Bite of a mad dog	47
— of a snake	264
Black cancer	265
Bladder, eversion of	159
— paralysis	160
— rupture	158
Blain	105
Bleeding	23
Blisters	21
Blood	26
— disorders, non-specific	64
— — specific	26
"Bloody" urine	70
Blunting teeth	45
Bone, cancer of	257
Bones	245
— feeding on	123
Bothriocephalus	136
Bowels	108
— diseases of	124

INDEX.

	PAGE		PAGE
Bowels, dropping of	128	Chorea	209
— inflammation, bilious of	142	Chorioptes	224
— parasites	131	Chronic bronchitis	95
— torpidity	115	— hepatitis	143
Brain	199	Cirrhosis testis	170
Break down	252	Circulatory disorders	73
Bright's disease	153	Circumcision	168
Broken teeth	100	Claws, mange of	254
Bronchitis	90	— overgrown	256
— chronic	95	— sinuous ulcer	255
— verminous	92	Cleft palate	104
Bronchocele	151	Clysters	17
Bug, harvest	238	Cold bath	23
		Colic	113
Cænurus	207	Condition, monstrous	193
Cæsarean operation	194	Congenital deformities	256
Calculus, biliary	147	— malformations	81
— cystic	156	— — penis	168
— intestinal	127	Congestion, pulmonary	97
— renal	154	Conjunctivitis	215
— urethral	164	— granular	215
Cancer	265	Constant desire	184
— bone	257	Constipation	115
— vagina	179	Consumption	62
Canine pathology	1	Copulation	166
— pharmacy	14	Cord, spinal	207
Canker, external	221	Cornea, opacity of	216
— internal	220	— ulceration of	216
— in mouth	103	Coryza	83
Cap for ears	222	Cramp	212
Capped elbow	266	Cracks on teats	198
— hock	266	Crochet	189
Carbolic acid	258	"Cropping"	220, 222
Carbonic acid poisoning	263	Curara	264
Caries of teeth	103	Cutaneous tuberculosis	229
Cartilago-nictitans tumours	215	Cutting the tushes	102
Castor-oil mixture	18	Cystic calculus	156
Castration	162	— growths	266
Cat epizooty (Delhi)	62	— hernia	159
Cataract	217	Cysticercus	136
Catarrh	83	Cystitis	156
— gastric	117	Cysts of retention	155
Cathartics	18		
Catheter	160	Deafness	220
— passage of	181	Death	263
Catheterism	160	Deformities, congenital	256
Causes of disease	7	Degeneration, fatty, heart	75
Cephalotomy	188	— liver	145
Chambers, nasal	82	Delayed parturition	187
Chances after bite of mad dog	48	Demodex	235
Changes, nutritive	72	Deposits on heart valves	73
Chest	89	Dermatitis	226
— founder	65	Dermatophytes	241
— inflammation of	90	Dermatozoa	230
Cheiracanthus	137	Dermoid tumours	217
Chloroforming	20	Destruction of dogs	263
Choking	108	Dew claws	256
Cholera	61	Diabetes mellitus	161

INDEX. 281

	PAGE		PAGE
Diagnosis of rabies	38	Ejecta, state of	10
Diaphragm, disorders of	97	Electric shock	263
— hernia of	97	Embryotomy	187
Diarrhœa	114	Emetics	19
Diet	12	Encephalitis	206
Digestive apparatus, disorders of	98	Enemata	17
		Enlargements, erectile, of penis	166
Dilatation, gastric	120	Enteritis	124
Diphtheria	56	Entropium	214
Disappearance of pancreas	149	Epilepsy	200
Diseases, dermatophytic	241	Epiplocele	130
— bowels	124	Epistaxis	86
— ductless glands	151	Erectile enlargements of penis	166
— liver	146	Ergot of rye	178
— prostatic	161	Erysipelas	229
— stomach	117	Erythema simplex	226
— tongue	104	Etherisation	21
Dislocation	250	Eustrongylus	155
— eyeball	218	Euthanasia	263
Disorders, circulatory	73	Eversis vesicæ	159
— blood, specific	26	Eye	214
— digestive apparatus	98	Eye changes in rabies	36
Displacement of teeth	101	Eyeball, dislocation of	218
— — liver	146	— extirpation of	218
— uterine	174	— trumatic distension of	217
Distemper	49	Eyelid, ulceration of	214
— putrid	55	Examination of dog patients	13
Distension of eyeball	217	— of foot	254
Distoma	146	Excision, spleen	150
Dochmius	133	— womb	177
Dog nuisance	7	Excretory apparatus, liver	147
Doses	21	Exercise	13
Double fœtus	193	Exostosis	252
Draughts	16	Expectorants	19
Dropping of bowel	128	External applications	21
Dropsy, aqueous	216	— canker	221
— brain	217	Extirpation of eyeball	218
— subcutaneous	229	Extractors	189, 190
— womb	173	Extra-uterine fœtation	193
Drowning	263		
Ductless glands	151		
Dumb madness	30	False conception	183
Dysentery	126	— joint	250
		— pains	185
		— tuberculosis	62
Ear	219	Fatty degeneration, heart	75
— ache	219	— liver	145
— cap	222	— tumours	266
— flap, scurfiness of	223	Favus	243
— polypi of	224	Feeding dogs on bones	123
Eating fœtal membranes	195	Feet, sore	254
— pups	195	Female genital organs	170
Eclampsia, puerperal	209	Femoral hernia	130
Ectopia hepatis	146	Fever	71
Ectropion	214	Fibroma	266
Eczema	226	Fibro-cystic tumours	266
— epizootica	58	Fibrous polypi	266
— mercuriale	259	Fighting dogs, to separate	267

	PAGE		PAGE
Filaria bepatica	146	Hæmorrhage, post-partum	178
— immitis	76	Hæmorrhagic tumours, spleen	150
— sanguinolenta	78, 108	Hæmorrboids	129
Firing	22	Harvest bug	238
Fistula, gastric	119	Head, injuries to	205
— biliary	147	Heart, degeneration of	75
— in ano	129	— rupture of	75
— lacteal	197	— valves, deposits on	73
Fits	200	— worms	76
Fleas	240	Hellebore	259
Fœtal appendages	193	Hepatitis	142
Fœtus, malposition of	185	— chronic	143
Fœtation extra-uterine	193	Hernia abdominalis	130
Follicular mange	235	— cystic	159
Fomentations	22	— diaphragmatic	97
Foot	253	— femoral	130
— examination of	254	— inguinal	130
— and-mouth disease	58	— uteri	174
Foreign bodies in stomach	120	— ventral	131
Forceps	189, 190	Holostoma	137
Foul	71	Honeycomb ringworm	243
Foulness of skin	226	Hornet stings	264
Foundered feet	254	Husk	117
Fractures	245	Hydatids	133, 136
Furious madness	209	— kidney	155
		Hydrocephalus	207
		Hydrocyanic acid	263
Gastric catarrh	117	Hydrometra	173
— dilatation	120	Hydropbobia, *vide* rabies.	
— fistula	119	Hydrops uteri	173
— intussusception	112	Hygiene of pregnancy	185
— ulcer	119	Hypersalivation	106
Gastritis	118	Hypertrophy, kidney	155
Gastro-bysterotomy	194	Hysterocele	174
General bebaviour	10		
— symptoms	8		
— — alimentary	111	Icterus	69
Generative apparatus	165, 170	Incisors	99
Genital organs, male	165	Impaction	127
Glanders	61	Impotence	169
Glands, ductless	151	Inappetance	111
Glans penis, inflammation of	167	Incontinence of urine	159
Glossitis	154	Indian arrow poison	264
Goitre	151	Indigestion	111
Gonorrbœa	163	Inertia uteri	178
Granular conjunctivitis	215	Infibulation	181
Growths, cystic	266	Infiltration, fatty, of heart	75
— malignant	197, 265	Inflammation of chest	90
— non-malignant	266	— of iris and choroid	219
— osseous	266	— of scrotum	168
— warty	167, 198, 266	Influences, nervous	11
Gullet, diseases of	108	Influenza	49
Gunsbot wounds	267	Inguinal hernia	130
		Imperforate prepuce	168
Hæmatemesis	119	Injection, subcutaneous	16, 21
Hæmatoma	223	Injuries to head	205
Hæmatozoa	76	Intestines	108
Hæmaturia	160	Inoculation for rabies	42

INDEX.

	PAGE
Intellect, aberrations of	200
Interference operations in parturition	187
Internal canker	220
— temperature	10
Intestines, diseases of	124
Intussusception	127
— gastric	112
Invagination	127
Inversio uteri	176
— vaginæ	180
Iris and choroid, inflammation of	219
Ixodes	240
Jaundice	69
Jaw, abscess of	103
Joint, false	250
— stiff	252
Kennel lameness	66
"Kernels"	151
Kidneys	158
Laceration, ligament, supra-orbital	215
— trapezius	252
— vagina	178
Lachrymal obstruction	215
Lactation	196
Lacteal fistula	197
Laparotomy	127, 137
Laryngitis	88
Laryngismus stridulus	88
Lead-poisoning	263
Leptus autumnalis	238
Leucorrhœa	180
Leukæmia	68
Lice	241
Ligament, supra-orbital, laceration of	215
Lips	98
— ulceration of	107
Lithotrity, natural	158
Liver	140
— abscess	143
— degenerations	145
— excretory apparatus	147
— rupture of	145
Lochia	195
"Locking"	166
Locomotor ataxia	209
— apparatus	245
Looseness of bowels	114
Loss of molars	104
— — voice	87
Lumbago	65
Lungs	89

	PAGE
Madness, dumb	30
— furious	29
Maggots	267
Male genital organs	165
Malformations, congenital	81
— — penis	168
Malignant growths	197
— disease, liver	146
— — ovaries	171
— — spleen	151
— tumours	265
— variola	60
Malingerers	11
Malposition of fœtus	185
Mammary concretions	196
— glands	196
— tumours	198
Mammitis	197
Mange of claw	254
— follicular	235
— red	228, 232
— true	230
Master MacGrath	81, 199
Materia medica	17, 269
Measles	61
Medicines	17, 269
Melanosis	265
Membrana pupillaris, persistence of	219
Menier's disease	224
Mercury compound	259
Metritis	172
Micorimyces	265
Milk	196
— abscess	196
Minor surgery	21, 264
Mixture, castor-oil	18
Molars	100
— loss of	104
Moles	193
— canker	103
Mouth, warts in	107
Monsters	193
Morbid appetite, bitch	195
Mouth	98
Morgagni's sinuses	129
Mucous membranes	10
Muzzle	21
Muzzling	24
Maw-worms	132
Narcotics	20
Nasal chambers	82
— polypus	86
Natal callosities	266
Natural lithotrity	158
Neck of bladder, stricture of	159

INDEX.

	PAGE		PAGE
Nephritis	154	Parasitic bronchitis	92
— albuminous	153	— disease, liver	146
Nerve grafting	213	— ozæna	85
Nervous influence	11	Parturient apoplexy	204
— system	199	Parturition	181, 185
Neuralgia	199	— assisted	186
Neurotomy	213	— delayed	187
Newly-born pup	193	— premature	186
Non-malignant growths	266	Passage of catheter	181
Non-specific blood diseases	64	Pasteur's researches	37, 42
Nursing	12	Pediculi	241
Nutritive changes	72	Penis, amputation of	168
		— bone	165
		Penien	165
Obstruction, lachrymal duct	215	Pentastoma	85
Œsophagotomy	110	Pericardial diseases	76
Œsophagus	107	Periostitis	257
— diseases of	108	Peritoueum	137
— stricture of	80	Peritonitis	137
Œstrum	181	Persistent membrana pupillaris	219
Olulanus	123	— vomition	112
Opacity of cornea	216	Pharmacy, canine	14
Operative interference, parturition	187	Pharyngitis	107
		Physiognomy of disease	8
Ophthalmia, simplex	215	Piles	29
Opisthotonos	212	Pills, administration of	14
Orchitis	170	Pityriasis	227
Organs of special sense	214	Placebos	10
Os penis	165	Plethora	71
Osseous growths	266	Pleurisy	90
Ostitis	219, 257	Pleurisy, worm	80
Ovaries	170	Pleurosthotonos	212
— atrophy of	171	Pneumonia	90
Ovariotomy	170	Poisoning	258
Overgrown claws	256	Polypi, fibrous	266
Overworn feet	254	— of ear	224
Ozæna	84	— of sheath	167
— parasitica	85	Polypus nasi	86
		— recti	130
		— vaginæ	179
Pachymeningitis, spinal	209	Posthitis	163, 167
Pads of feet	254	Post-partum hæmorrhage	178
Pains, false	185	Pregnancy	184
Palate	98	— hygiene	185
— cleft	104	Premature parturition	186
Pancreas	140, 148	Prolapsus ani	128
— disappearance of	149	— recti	128
Paracentesis abdominis	139	— vaginæ	180
Paralysis	207	Prepuce, imperforate	168
— bladder	160	Profuse staling	160
— tongue	104	Prolapsus uteri	176
Paraplegia, worm	80	Prostatic disease	161
Parasites, brain	207	Prussic acid	263
— renal	155	Psoriasis	227
— stomach	122	Ptyalism	106
— toes	256	Puerperal eclampsia	209
— urethral	164	Pulex	240
Parasitic affections, skin	229	Pulmonary apoplexy	97

INDEX. 285

	PAGE		PAGE
Pulmonary congestion	97	Sinuses, facial	82
Pulse	8	— of Morgagni	129
Pup, newly-born	193	Sinuous ulcer, claw	255
Purgatives	18	Skin	225
Putrid distemper	56	— foulness of	226
		Skunk bite	44
Rabies	26	Snake bite	264
— inoculation	42	Snoring	87
Rachitis	67	Snorting	86
Ranula	106	Sore feet	254
Rasping of tushes	102	Sore throat	84
Rectal diseases	128	Spaying	170
Red mange	228, 232	Spavins	252
Relapsing fever	58	Special sense organs	214
Relation of canine to human		Specific blood disorders	26
disorders	13	Spermatic cord	170
Renal calculus	154	Spinal cord	207
— parasites	155	— pachymeningitis	209
Renitis	154	Spirilloids	58
Respirations	10	Spiroptera	123
Respiratory system	82	Spleen	140, 149
Retention cysts	155	— excision of	150
— of milk	196	— ruptured	150
— — urine	159	— tumours	150
Rheumatism	64	Splenic apoplexy	151
Rickets	66	Splenitis	149
Ringworm	242	Splints	252
— honeycomb	243	Sprains	252
Round-worms	132	Staling, profuse	160
"Rounding"	222	Staphyloma	216
Rupture of bladder	158	Stiff joints	252
— — heart	75	Stimulants	20
— — liver	145	Stings	264
— — spleen	150	Stomach	107
— — stomach	120	— disease of	117
		— foreign bodies in	120
		— parasites in	122
Sacculus, intestinal	127	— pump	16
St. Vitus's dance	209	— ruptured	120
Sarcoma	265	Strangury	159
— spleen	151	Stricture, neck of bladder	159
Sarcoptes canis	231	— bowel	130
Sarcoptic scabies	230	— œsophagus	80, 108
Scabies, sarcoptic	230	Strongylus canis bronchialis	94
Scantiness of urine	159	— gigas	164
Scrotum, inflammation of	168	— vasorum	62
Scurfiness of ear-flap	228	Strychnia	262
Sedatives	20	Sturdy in sheep	133
Sediments, urinary	161	Subcutaneous syringe	16
Seizure of mad dogs	39	Suckling of pups by women	196
Septicæmia	64	Superfœtation	183
Sero-sanguineous abscess ear-flap	228	Superpurgation	114
Sense organs, special	214	Suppression of urine	159
Separation of fighting dogs	267	Supra-orbital ligament, laceration	215
Setons	22		
Sheath, polypi of	167	Surgery, minor	21, 264
Simple erythema	226	Surra	58
— ophthalmia	215	Symbiotes	231

	PAGE		PAGE
Symptoms, general	8	Tumours, dermoid	217
System, locomotor	245	— fatty	266
— nervous	199	— fibrocystic	266
— respiratory	82	— mammary	198
Subcutaneous tissue, dropsy of	229	— uterine	178
Sudoriparous glands	225	— vaginal	179
Surfeit	226	Tushes	100
		— cutting of	102
Tabes	63	Turnsick in sheep	133
Tæniæ	133, 136	Twist of the womb	175
Tæniafuges	19		
Tapeworms	133	Ulcer in stomach	119
"Tapping the belly"	139	Ulceration, cornea	216
Tartar accumulations	100	— eyelids	214
Teats, diseases of	198	— lips	107
Teeth	99	— womb	172
— blunting of	46	Unicity	61
— broken	101	Urethral calculus	164
— displacement of	101	— diseases	164
— excessive wear of	101	— parasites	164
Temperature, internal	10	Urinary apparatus	153
Tenotomy	257	Urination, abnormal	159
Testes, diseases of	170	Urine	160
Tetanus	212	— incontinence of	159
Toes, amputation of	256	— retention of	159
— parasites of	256	— scantiness of	159
Tongue	98	— suppression of	159
Thorn wounds of foot	256	Uterine dropsy	173
Throat forceps	110	— displacements	174
Thymus body	152	— inertia	178
Thyroid body	151	— prolapsus	176
Ticks	240	— tumour	178
— in ear	223	Uterus	172
Tinea favosa	243	— amputation of	177
— tonsurans	242	Ureter	155
Tobacco water	259	Urethritis	163
Tougue, diseases of	104		
— paralysis of	104	Vaccination for anthrax	59
— wounds of	105	Vagina, laceration of	178
Torpidity of bowels	115	— prolapsus of	180
Torsio uteri	175	— tumours of	179
Toxicology	258	Valves of heart, diseases of	73
Traumatic distension of eyeball	217	Variola	60
Treatment	10	Vegetable poisoning	260
Trichina	133	Venesection	23
Trichocephalus	133	Ventral hernia	131
Trichodectes latus	133	Vermifuges	19
Trichophyton tonsurans	242	Verminous bronchitis	92
— favosa	243	Verrucæ	229
Trichisis	214	Vertigo	201
True mange	230	Voice, loss of	87
— fracture	245	Volvulus	127
Trapezius, laceration of	252	Vomition	112
Tuberculosis	62	— persistent	112
— cutaneous	229		
— false	62	Warm bath	22
Tumours	265	Washing	13, 23
— cartilago nictitans	215	"Watery eye"	214

Warts 229	Worms in heart . . . 76
— in mouth 107	"Worming" 98
Warty growths . . . 167, 266	Wounds 267
— growths teats . . . 198	— punctured pericardium . 76
Wasps' stings 264	— thorn-foot 256
Wear, excessive, of teeth . . 101	— tongue 105
Womb 172	Wourali 264
— excision of 177	
Worms in bowels . . . 131	"Yellows" 69

www.ingramcontent.com/pod-product-compliance
Lightning Source LLC
Chambersburg PA
CBHW021623250426
43672CB00037B/1358